LIFESAVERS

THE COMPLETE HOME MEDICAL & EMERGENCY HANDBOOK

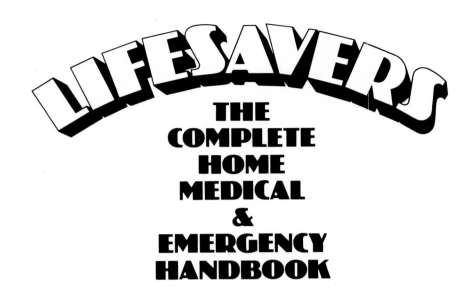

LIFESAVERS

THE COMPLETE HOME MEDICAL & EMERGENCY HANDBOOK

Created, Designed and Produced
by
Martin I. Green

BALLANTINE BOOKS • NEW YORK

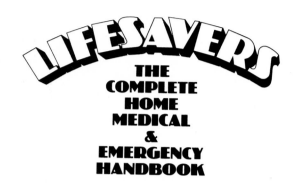

LIFESAVERS
THE COMPLETE HOME MEDICAL & EMERGENCY HANDBOOK

Copyright © 1981 by Martin I. Green
Library of Congress Catalog Card Number: 81-67559
ISBN: 0-345-29032-1

Published in the United States by Ballantine Books, a division of Random House, Inc., New York, and simultaneously in Canada by Random House of Canada, Limited, Toronto, Canada.

This edition published by arrangement with Martin I. Green and Berkshire Studio.
Manufactured in the United States of America
First Edition: MARCH 1982
135798642

CREDITS

Created, Designed & Produced by	MARTIN I. GREEN
Edited by	ROSS FIRESTONE
Illustrator & Associate Designer	BOBBI BONGARD
Research	
Part One: Emergencies & Mishaps	PAUL A. CIRINCIONE
Part Two: Illnesses & Disorders	LAWRENCE GALTON
Editorial Assistant	BERNICE CIRINCIONE
Proofreader	CIA ELKIN
Mechanical Art	CANDY SEYLER
Inspiration	MARY & JARED GREEN

Many thanks to Ben Schawinsky and Herbert Sipp for
their help and assistance. Thanks, too, to Donna M. Albano, Michael J. Albano,
George Angermann, Seymour Z. Baum, Frank Bongard, Madeline Bongard,
Nancy Coffey, Ken Curtiss, Martha Donovan, Noah Elkin, Samson Elkin,
Gail Firestone, Simon Firestone, Stephen Kaufman, Patrick Montoir,
Nancy Neiman, J. Christopher Procopio, Joanne Brouwer Procopio,
The Stockpot, John Zito and Russel Zito.

A very special thanks to Leonard Rubin for his friendship and brilliance.
I will always miss him.   MIG

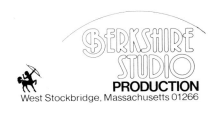

Berkshire Studio
PRODUCTION
West Stockbridge, Massachusetts 01266

ACKNOWLEDGMENTS

We wish to thank the following for providing us with information, for making their facilities available to us, and for reviewing and commenting on the manuscript during its various phases.

George Armstrong
Director
National Clearinghouse of Poison Control Centers
Rockville, Maryland

C. P. Dail
Director of First Aid Services
American Red Cross
National Headquarters
Washington, D.C.

Lawrence Lerman, M.D.
Chief, Division of General Medicine
The Mount Sinai Medical Center
Associate Chairman, Department of Medicine
The Mount Sinai School of Medicine
New York, New York

Norman Metzger
Vice President
The Mount Sinai Medical Center
Professor, Department of Health Care Management
The Mount Sinai School of Medicine
New York, New York

Don Sleeper
Assistant Director of First Aid Services
American Red Cross
National Headquarters
Washington, D.C.

Thanks, too, to the following for providing information and for their research on our behalf:

American Burn Association
University of Alabama
Birmingham, Alabama

American Cancer Society
New York, New York

American Diabetes Association
New York, New York

American Heart Association
Dallas, Texas

American Lung Association
New York, New York

Asthma & Allergy Foundation of America
New York, New York

Maryland Poison Information Center
Gary Oderda, Ph.D.
Baltimore, Maryland

Rocky Mountain Poison Center
John B. Sullivan Jr., M.D.
Denver, Colorado

University of Miami Medical School
Kenneth S. Lampe, Ph.D.
Miami, Florida

United States Coast Guard
John C. Bernhartsen
Washington, D.C.

United States Coast Guard
LCDR William R. Ladd
Washington, D.C.

FOR
MY FATHER
BEN GREEN
WITH MUCH LOVE
AND
APPRECIATION

CONTENTS

Introduction by Lawrence Lerman, M.D.

PART ONE
EMERGENCIES & MISHAPS: FIRST-AID PROCEDURES

PART TWO
ILLNESSES AND DISORDERS

INTRODUCTION

by Lawrence Lerman, M.D.

Chief, Division of General Medicine
The Mount Sinai Medical Center
Associate Chairman, Department of Medicine
The Mount Sinai School of Medicine
New York, New York

The past decade has witnessed a tremendous growth of concern about physical well-being in this country. Americans have significantly increased the time and effort devoted to exercise, athletics and outdoor recreational pursuits. We have become more conscious than ever of the importance of adequate nutrition and proper diet. These changes have brought with them a new awareness of the responsibility we all must take for preserving our own good health. Indeed, in recent years there has been a positive flood of programs and publications promoting self care. Many of these enterprises have been geared to the needs of highly specific subgroups — runners, the overweight, etc. What has been needed is a readable manual that is broad enough in content and approach to have relevance for the general population. **LIFESAVERS** fills this need by its treatment of family medical care, a subject — perhaps **the** subject — of primary concern to all of us, layman and medical professional alike.

The first section is a superb presentation of the emergency techniques necessary to preserve life and limb. Wisely, it also includes instructions on how to cope with minor (but by no means trivial) injuries and ailments. Unlike many of the other first-aid manuals now available, its format is specifically designed for use in an emergency situation, when every second counts and stress makes it difficult to extract crucial information from cumbersome paragraphs of fine print buried somewhere inside the text. The index on the back cover gives the reader-in-a-hurry immediate access to the appropriate first-aid procedure. The instructions are pared down to essentials and presented in direct, lucid, nontechnical language printed in easily read large type. They are supported by hundreds of illustrative graphics which add a specificity all to often missing from efforts of this kind. This clarity of presentation and lack of ambiguity attest to a creative blending of medical expertise and editorial skill.

A second section serves to explain a host of relatively common illnesses and disorders that flesh is heir to. In addition to providing good general information, these concise expositions of symptoms, causes and steps to be taken should help alert the reader to medical problems that might otherwise be overlooked or discounted in their early stages, when they are most responsive to treatment. The information included here can also provide the basis for a productive dialogue with one's personal physician.

I am impressed that this book has taken account of the fact that health care is a dynamic body of knowledge, in a constant state of adjustment and change. The list of acknowledgements clearly demonstrates that every effort has been made to obtain a consensus of leading experts in emergency care and health management so as to provide the most up-to-date information and techniques.

LIFESAVERS belongs in the home, car, vacation spot and anywhere else that family members congregate.

PART ONE

EMERGENCIES & MISHAPS: FIRST-AID PROCEDURES

FIRST-AID SUPPLIES

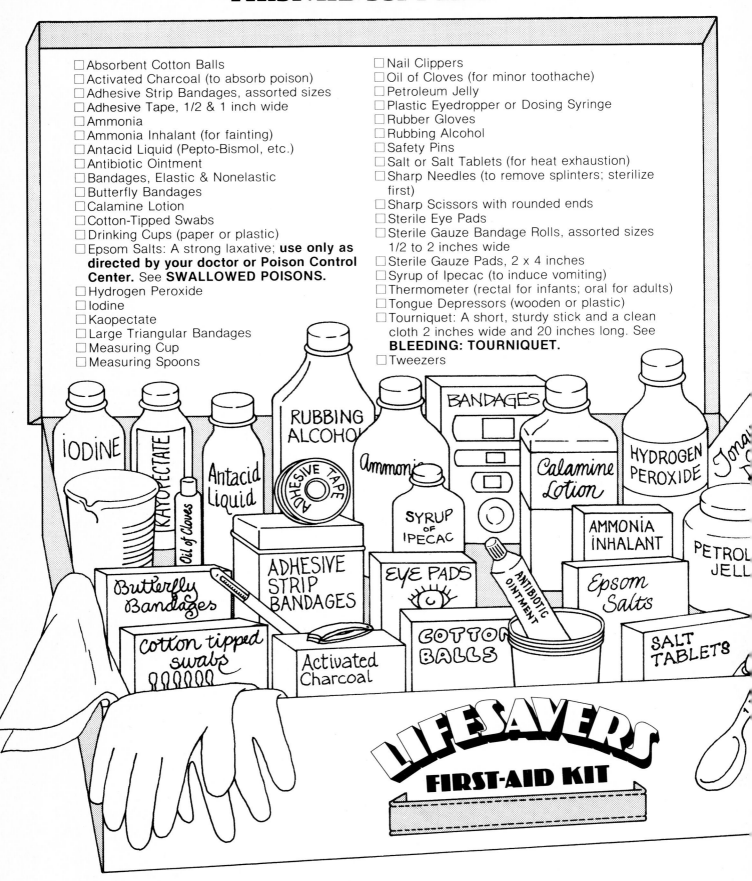

- ☐ Absorbent Cotton Balls
- ☐ Activated Charcoal (to absorb poison)
- ☐ Adhesive Strip Bandages, assorted sizes
- ☐ Adhesive Tape, 1/2 & 1 inch wide
- ☐ Ammonia
- ☐ Ammonia Inhalant (for fainting)
- ☐ Antacid Liquid (Pepto-Bismol, etc.)
- ☐ Antibiotic Ointment
- ☐ Bandages, Elastic & Nonelastic
- ☐ Butterfly Bandages
- ☐ Calamine Lotion
- ☐ Cotton-Tipped Swabs
- ☐ Drinking Cups (paper or plastic)
- ☐ Epsom Salts: A strong laxative; **use only as directed by your doctor or Poison Control Center.** See **SWALLOWED POISONS.**
- ☐ Hydrogen Peroxide
- ☐ Iodine
- ☐ Kaopectate
- ☐ Large Triangular Bandages
- ☐ Measuring Cup
- ☐ Measuring Spoons

- ☐ Nail Clippers
- ☐ Oil of Cloves (for minor toothache)
- ☐ Petroleum Jelly
- ☐ Plastic Eyedropper or Dosing Syringe
- ☐ Rubber Gloves
- ☐ Rubbing Alcohol
- ☐ Safety Pins
- ☐ Salt or Salt Tablets (for heat exhaustion)
- ☐ Sharp Needles (to remove splinters; sterilize first)
- ☐ Sharp Scissors with rounded ends
- ☐ Sterile Eye Pads
- ☐ Sterile Gauze Bandage Rolls, assorted sizes 1/2 to 2 inches wide
- ☐ Sterile Gauze Pads, 2 x 4 inches
- ☐ Syrup of Ipecac (to induce vomiting)
- ☐ Thermometer (rectal for infants; oral for adults)
- ☐ Tongue Depressors (wooden or plastic)
- ☐ Tourniquet: A short, sturdy stick and a clean cloth 2 inches wide and 20 inches long. See **BLEEDING: TOURNIQUET.**
- ☐ Tweezers

SPECIAL KITS AVAILABLE

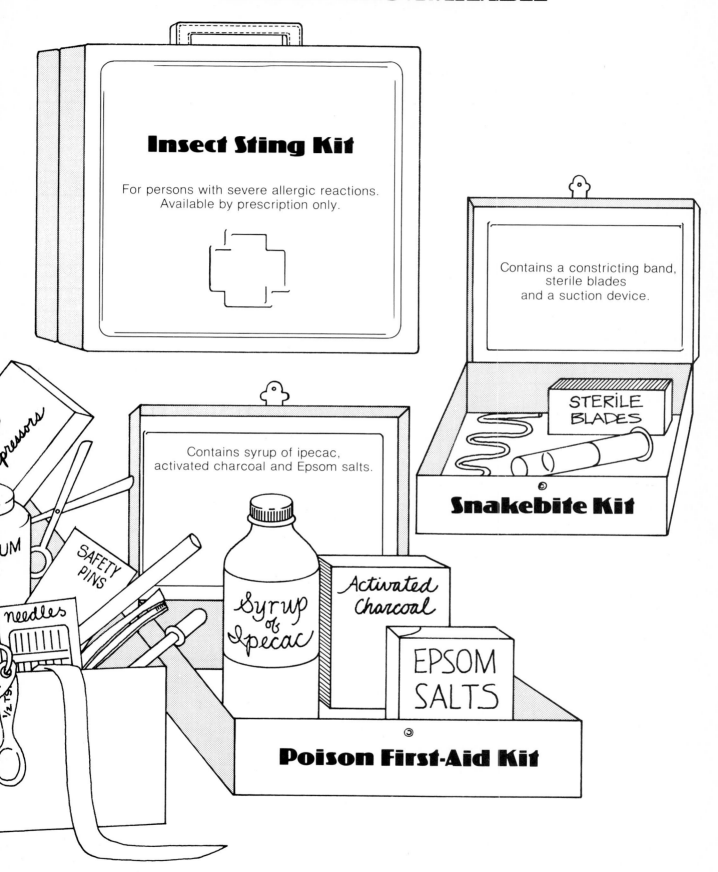

Insect Sting Kit

For persons with severe allergic reactions.
Available by prescription only.

Contains a constricting band,
sterile blades
and a suction device.

STERILE BLADES

Snakebite Kit

Contains syrup of ipecac,
activated charcoal and Epsom salts.

Syrup of Ipecac

Activated Charcoal

EPSOM SALTS

SAFETY PINS

needles

Poison First-Aid Kit

First aid is not a substitute for professional medical care. If someone in your household becomes seriously injured or ill, you should always try to obtain the immediate assistance of a physician. Unfortunately, this isn't always possible. Emergencies have a way of happening when help isn't available right away, and if they aren't dealt with promptly the victim's life may be jeopardized. Under such circumstances, your ability to provide quick, effective first aid may mean the difference between life and death.

This section presents the most up-to-date first-aid procedures for all the common emergencies you are most likely to encounter. It also includes instructions on how to handle such common mishaps as splinters and blisters. To help you act quickly and correctly, each procedure combines clear, simple instructions printed in large type with easy to follow step-by-step illustrations. As a further help, the back cover of this book is thumb-indexed to give you immediate access to the procedures for the most serious emergencies. Each procedure is also listed in the **CONTENTS** in the front of the book.

There are several crucial points to keep in mind whenever you have to come to someone's aid:

• It is, of course, terribly distressing to see a loved one suffering from an illness or injury, but if you are to alleviate the emergency you must do your best to remain calm and clearheaded so you can follow the appropriate procedures correctly.

• If you are unsure about the nature or extent of an emergency, see **ASSESSING THE EMERGENCY** before attempting any first aid. There are times when doing the incorrect thing can be more injurious than not doing anything at all. Hippocrates articulated the principle when he said, "First, do no harm."

We suggest you read through this section as soon as possible to familiarize yourself with the recommended procedures before you ever need to use them. Remember that the basic purpose of first aid is to preserve the victim's life and prevent further physical and psychological harm until help arrives. We also suggest that you keep this book in an accessible place known to everyone in your family.

To obtain the best possible preparation for medical emergencies, sign up for the first-aid courses offered by your local chapter of the **American National Red Cross.** The basic and advanced programs provide training and supervised practice in virtually every aspect of emergency care. **Special training for cardiopulmonary resuscitation (CPR), the first-aid technique for heart failure, is especially important; the procedure can cause serious harm if used unnecessarily or incorrectly.**

With the proper foresight, many medical emergencies can be prevented altogether. The **National Safety Council** has developed a great variety of preventive techniques applicable to all ages and activities. You can obtain this information by writing the National Safety Council at 444 North Michigan Avenue, Chicago, Illinois 60611.

IMPORTANT

- **If the situation seems at all serious, send for medical aid immediately.**

- **Do not move the person unless it is absolutely necessary.** You may cause further harm.

- **If unconscious, do not** give the person anything to drink.

- Try to get an account of what happened. Ask the victim or bystanders who may have witnessed the event.

- Check the victim for medical information tags or cards.

- Treat the most serious injuries first.

- Remain calm and offer reassurance and comfort.

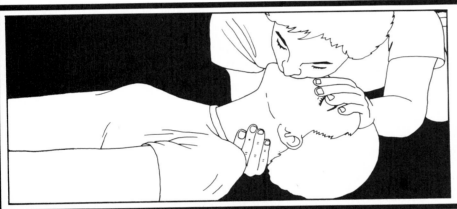

1 If unconscious, check the person's breathing. If necessary, see **BREATHING: ARTIFICIAL RESPIRATION.**

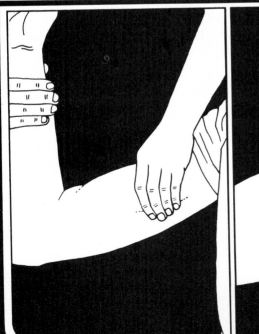
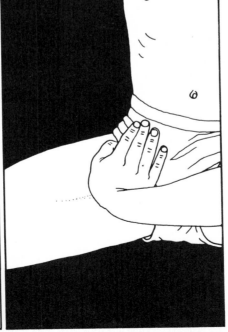

2 **Check for bleeding.** Quickly and gently examine the head and body for injuries. Make sure not to overlook any concealed wounds. Control the most serious bleeding first. See **BLEEDING: CUTS & WOUNDS.**

CONTINUED ON NEXT PAGE

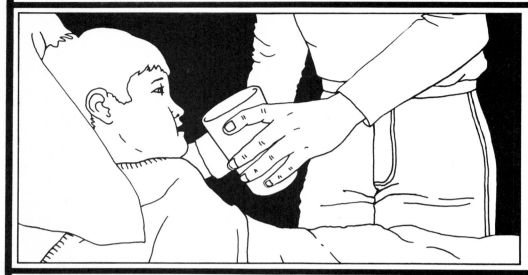

3 If there are burns or stains on the mouth or other signs of poisoning (pills, chemicals, etc.), see **POISONING.**

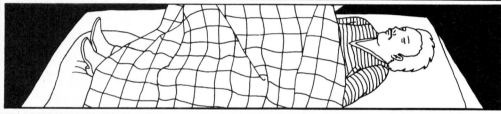

4 Observe for shock; see **SHOCK.**

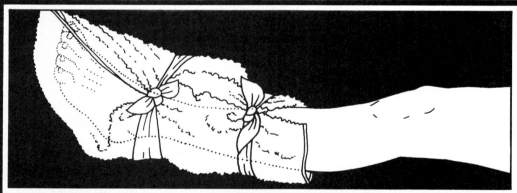

5 For broken bones, see **BREAKS: FRACTURES & DISLOCATIONS.**

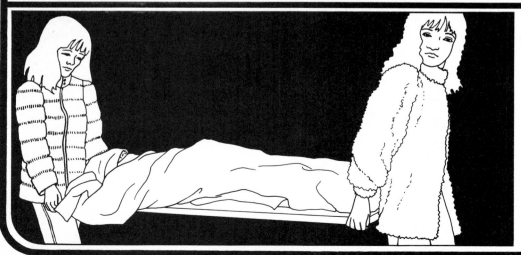

6 In cool or cold weather, particularly if it is windy and the person is wet, see **HYPOTHERMIA.**

ABRASIONS

- **Seek medical aid immediately** if an eye or a large area of the body is affected, if dirt or foreign substances have been ground into the wound or if there is evidence of infection. **Do not** treat these abrasions yourself.

SYMPTOMS

Surface of the skin is scraped, scratched or rubbed away. Reddening of the affected area. May or may not bleed, depending on severity.

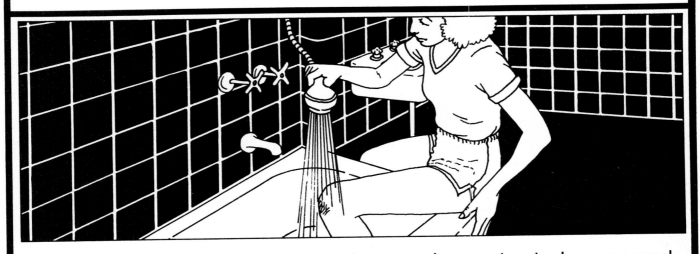

1 Place the affected area under running water to loosen and wash away dirt. If necessary, gently remove foreign matter with a sterile gauze pad or clean cloth.

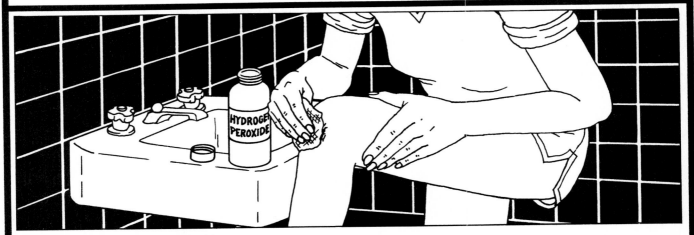

2 Wash the affected area with hydrogen peroxide or soap and water.

CONTINUED ON NEXT PAGE

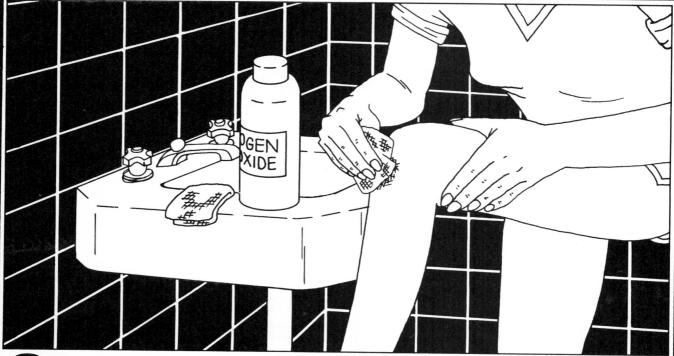

3 Gently blot dry with sterile gauze or a clean cloth.

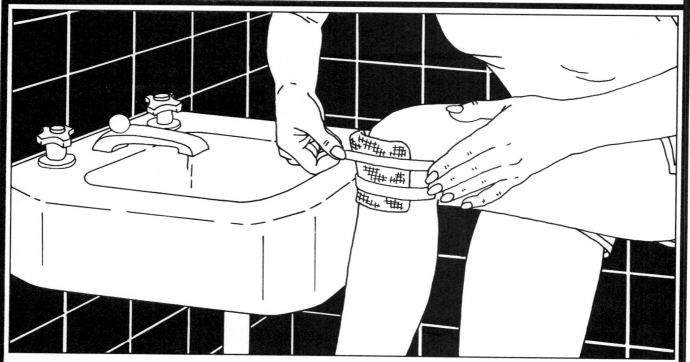

4 Cover with a clean, nonadhering dressing or cloth. Hold it in place with adhesive tape.

ASTHMA ATTACK

IMPORTANT

- **Seek medical aid** if the attack is severe or occurring for the first time.

- Watch breathing closely. If necessary, see **BREATHING: ARTIFICIAL RESPIRATION.**

- Someone with a history of asthma should avoid known or suspected causes of attacks.

SYMPTOMS

In early stages: Respiratory discomfort resembling a cold. Coughing. Nasal congestion. **May progress to:** Labored breathing with whistling or wheezing sounds. Anxiety. **In advanced cases:** Feeling of suffocation. Pale or bluish lips, gums, skin and fingernails. **May progress to:** Respiratory failure.

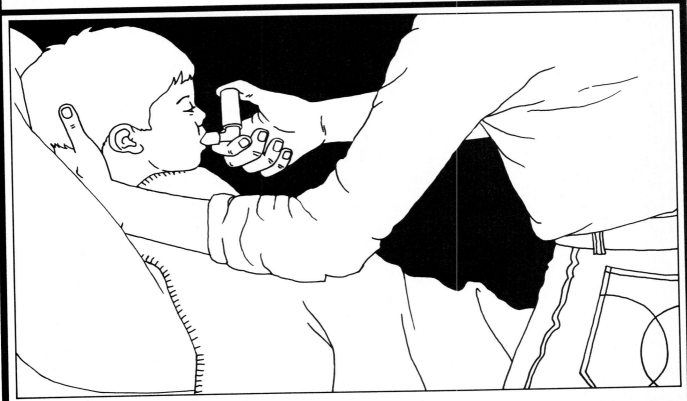

1 As soon as symptoms are noticed, take the person to a quiet area and place him in the most comfortable position: seated, semi-reclining or reclining. Provide good ventilation. If medicine has been prescribed, help the person take it.

CONTINUED ON NEXT PAGE

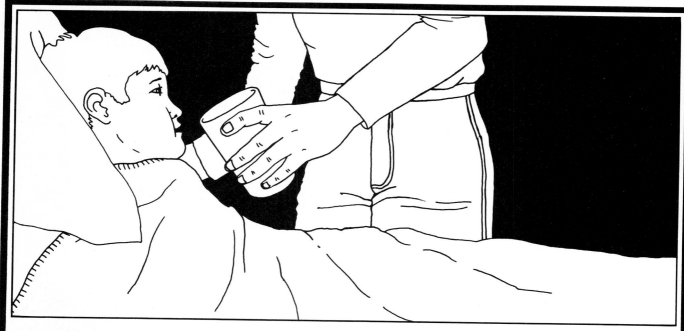

2 Have the person rest. Comfort and reassure him; anxiety may worsen the attack. Encourage him to drink plenty of liquids — water, fruit juices, etc. but not milk.

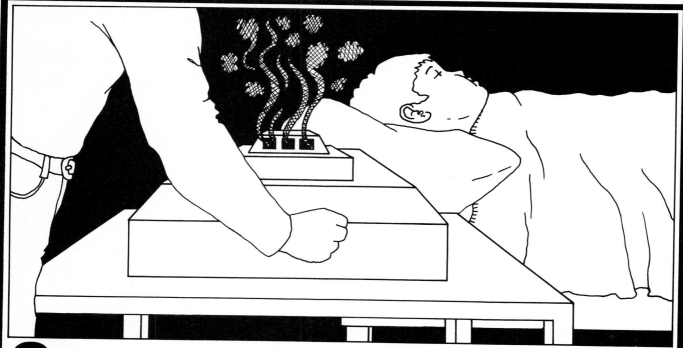

3 A cool-mist vaporizer may help ease distressed breathing.

IMPORTANT

- **Seek medical aid immediately.**

- **Do not** bend or twist the neck or body.

- **Do not** move the person unless you absolutely must. If it does become necessary, see **TRANSPORTING THE INJURED.**

- If the person has trouble breathing, see **BREATHING: ARTIFICIAL RESPIRATION.**

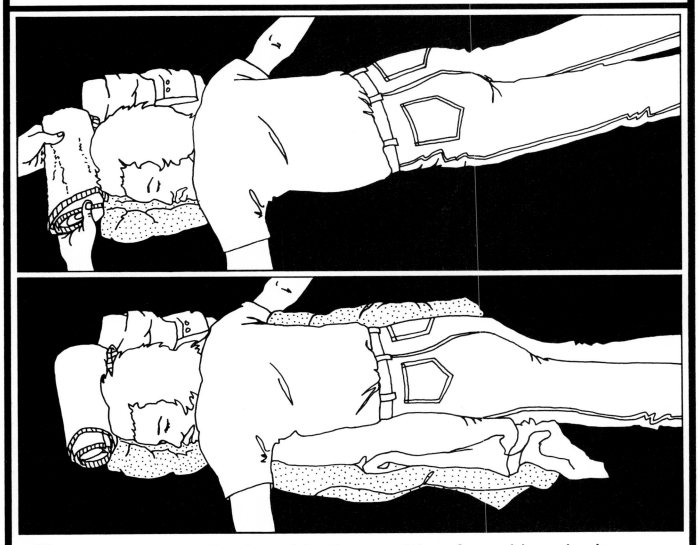

1A Immobilize the head in the position found by placing rolled up clothing, blankets, etc. around the head and the sides of the neck and shoulders. For back injuries, also immobilize the torso.

CONTINUED ON NEXT PAGE

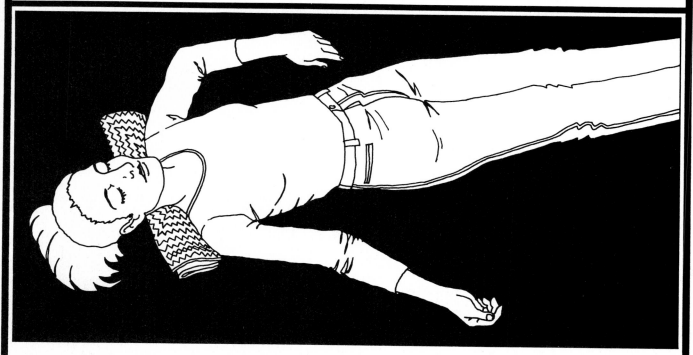

1B If the person is on her back, slide a small towel or pad under her neck without moving her head. (**Do not** place anything bulky under the head.)

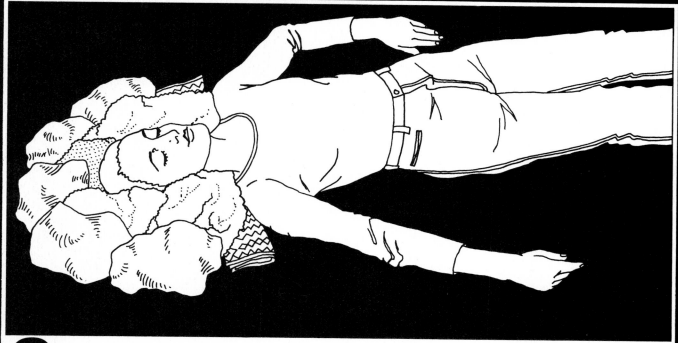

2 Hold restraining materials in place with bricks, stones, etc.

BITES & STINGS

ANIMAL & HUMAN BITES

IMPORTANT

- **If the skin is penetrated, seek medical aid immediately.** Human bites can be particularly dangerous.
- Try to capture or confine the animal for examination. Be careful not to get bitten yourself.
- Observe for shock; see **SHOCK.**

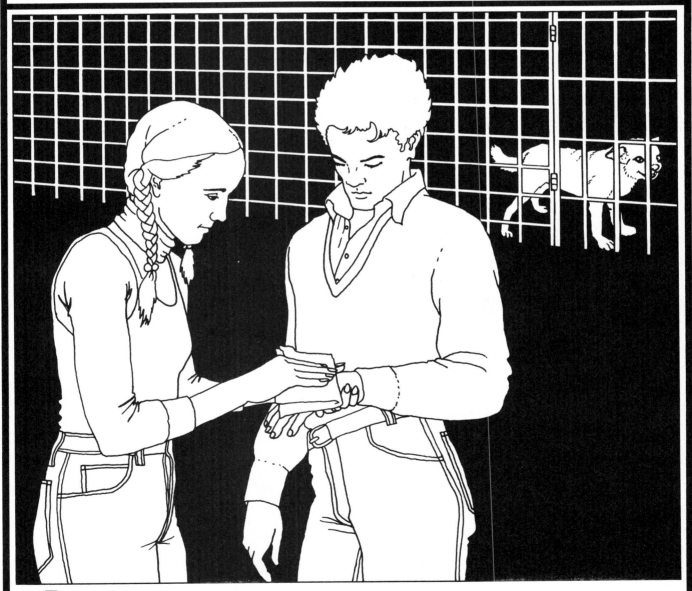

1 Control the bleeding. See **BLEEDING: CUTS & WOUNDS.**

CONTINUED ON NEXT PAGE

ANIMAL & HUMAN BITES
CONTINUED

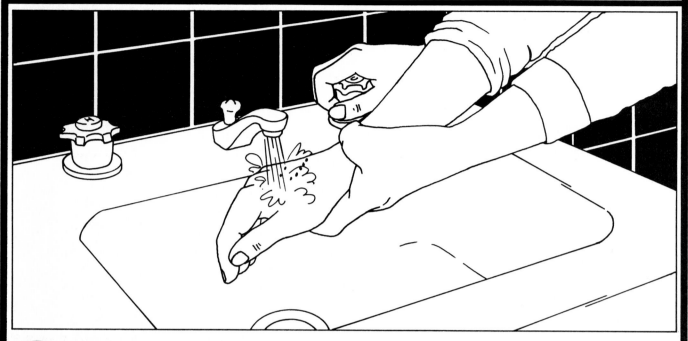

2 Wash the wound with soap and water. **Do not** use antiseptics, ointments or other medications.

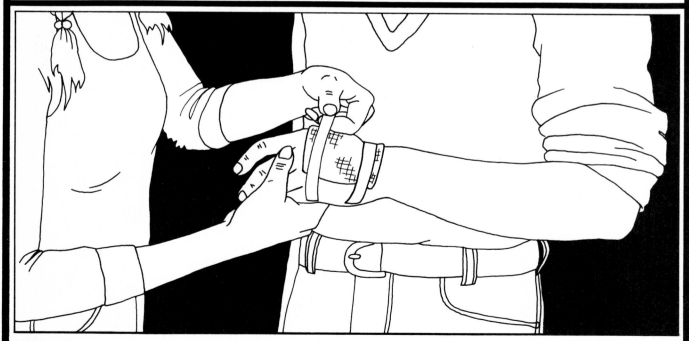

3 Apply a sterile dressing or clean cloth. Hold it in place with a bandage.

BITES & STINGS

INSECTS

IMPORTANT

- **Seek medical aid immediately** for bites and stings from **BLACK WIDOW** and **BROWN RECLUSE SPIDERS, SCORPIONS** and **TARANTULAS,** particularly if the person is subject to hay fever, asthma or any allergic reactions. Also observe for shock; see **SHOCK.**

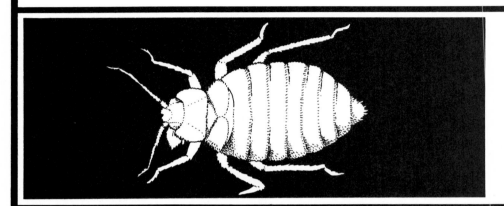

BEDBUG

SYMPTOMS: Welts. Swelling. Irritation.

WHAT TO DO: Wash thoroughly with soap and water.

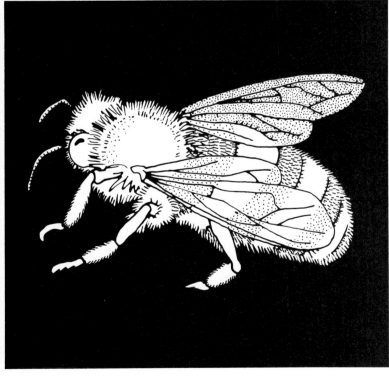

BEE (WASP, HORNET & YELLOW JACKET)

NOTE: Seek medical aid immediately if the person is subject to allergic reactions or if there is severe swelling anywhere on his body. Also observe for shock; see **SHOCK.** Watch breathing closely. If necessary, see **BREATHING: ARTIFICIAL RESPIRATION.**

SYMPTOMS: Pain. Local swelling. Burning and itching. Allergic reaction will also cause nausea, shock, unconsciousness and severe swelling.

WHAT TO DO: For a beesting, remove the venom sac by scraping gently, not by squeezing. (Wasps, hornets and yellow jackets do not leave venom sacs.) Wash with soap and water. For severe reactions, see first aid for **BLACK WIDOW SPIDER.**

CONTINUED ON NEXT PAGE

BITES & STINGS

INSECTS
CONTINUED

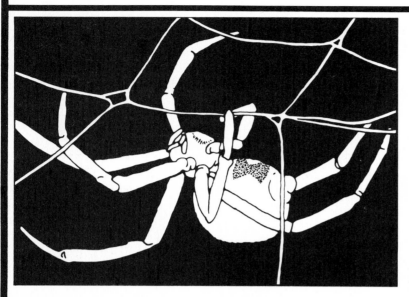

BLACK WIDOW SPIDER

SYMPTOMS: Severe pain. Profuse sweating. Muscle cramps. Difficulty breathing. Nausea.

WHAT TO DO: Watch breathing closely. If it stops, see **BREATHING: ARTIFICIAL RESPIRATION.** Keep the person quiet and avoid unnecessary movement. Keep the affected part below heart level. Place a constricting band 2 to 4 inches above the wound. **Do not** bind too tightly. You should be able to slide your finger under the band. Apply ice wrapped in a cloth. Remove the band after 30 minutes.

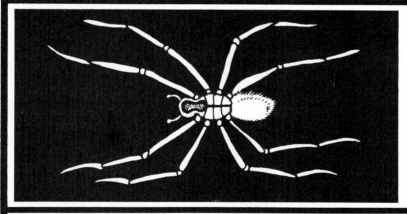

BROWN RECLUSE SPIDER

SYMPTOMS: The bite may be hardly noticed, but hours later severe pain, swelling and blisters occur.

WHAT TO DO: Follow first aid for **BLACK WIDOW SPIDER.**

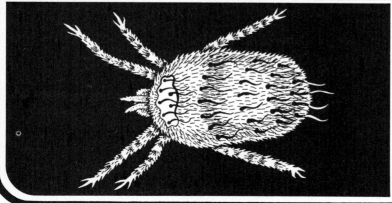

CHIGGER

SYMPTOMS: Itching. Irritation. Local pain. Small red welts.

WHAT TO DO: Wash with soap and water. Soothe irritation with cold compresses or calamine lotion.

BITES & STINGS

INSECTS

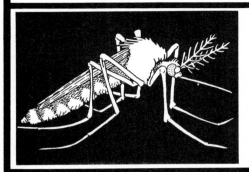

MOSQUITO

SYMPTOMS: Itching. Irritation. Local pain. Small red welts.

WHAT TO DO: Wash with soap and water. Soothe irritation with cold compresses or calamine lotion.

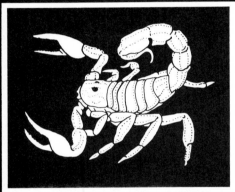

SCORPION

SYMPTOMS: Excruciating pain at the sting. Swelling. Fever. Nausea. Stomach pains. Difficulty speaking. Worsening convulsions. Coma.

WHAT TO DO: Follow first aid for **BLACK WIDOW SPIDER.**

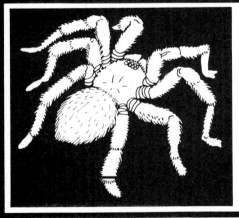

TARANTULA

SYMPTOMS: May vary from pinprick to severe wound.

WHAT TO DO: Wash with soap and water. Cover lightly with a sterile dressing or clean cloth. For severe reactions, see first aid for **BLACK WIDOW SPIDER.**

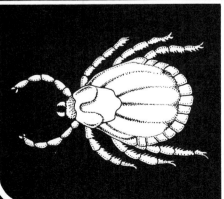

TICK

SYMPTOMS: The tick may be visible on the skin as a dark spot.

WHAT TO DO: Do not pull the tick from the person's skin. Apply heavy oil to the area, then after 30 minutes remove the parts of the tick carefully with a tweezer. Wash with soap and water.

BITES & STINGS

MARINE LIFE

- **Seek medical aid immediately.**
- Watch breathing closely. If necessary, see **BREATHING: ARTIFICIAL RESPIRATION.**
- Observe for shock; see **SHOCK.**

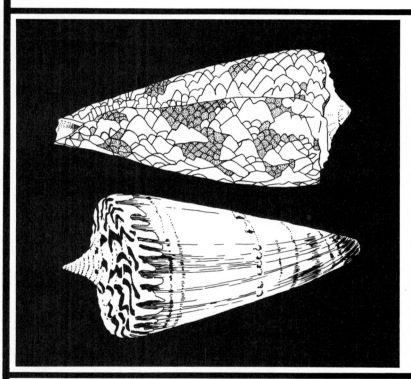

CONE SHELL

SYMPTOMS: Vary from a slight sting to severe pain, numbness, tingling, difficulty swallowing, tightness in the chest, partial paralysis, impaired vision, collapse.

WHAT TO DO: Place a constricting band 2 to 4 inches above the wound. **Do not** bind too tightly. You should be able to slide your finger under the band. Soak in hot water or apply hot compresses for 30 minutes, then remove the band.

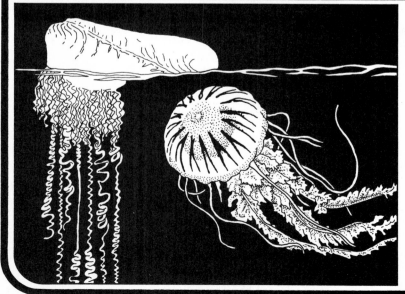

MAN-OF-WAR & JELLYFISH

SYMPTOMS: Burning pain. Rash. Swelling. Difficulty breathing. Cramps. Nausea. Vomiting. Collapse.

WHAT TO DO: Gently remove the tentacles with a cloth. Clean affected area with alcohol or with ammonia diluted with an equal amount of water.

BITES & STINGS

MARINE LIFE

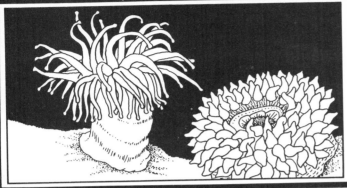

SEA ANEMONE & HYDROID

SYMPTOMS: Burning or stinging pain. Stomach cramps. Chills. Diarrhea.

WHAT TO DO: Soak in hot water or apply hot compresses.

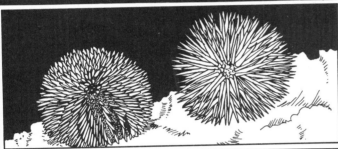

SEA URCHIN

SYMPTOMS: Pain. Dizziness. Muscle tremors. Paralysis.

WHAT TO DO: Apply a constricting band; see first aid for **CONE SHELL.**

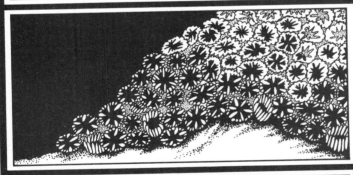

STINGING CORAL

SYMPTOMS: Burning or stinging pain.

WHAT TO DO: Wash thoroughly with soap and water.

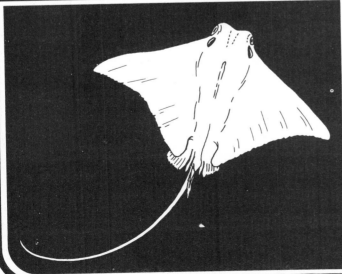

STINGRAY

SYMPTOMS: Painful cut or puncture. Swelling. Discoloration. Nausea. Vomiting. Muscle spasms. Convulsions. Difficulty breathing.

WHAT TO DO: Carefully remove the stinger if possible. Wash thoroughly with soap and water. Control the bleeding; see **BLEEDING: CUTS & WOUNDS.** Apply a constricting band; see first aid for **CONE SHELL.**

BITES & STINGS

SNAKEBITE

IMPORTANT

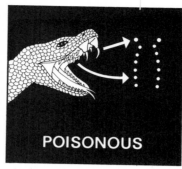
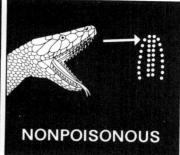

POISONOUS   NONPOISONOUS

- To determine if the bite is from a poisonous snake, look for fang marks at the wound. If nonpoisonous, see Step 4 only.

- **Seek medical aid immediately** for any snakebite or suspected snakebite.

- **Do not** let the person walk or move the affected part unless absolutely necessary.

- Keep the affected part below heart level.

- Watch breathing closely. If necessary, see **BREATHING: ARTIFICIAL RESPIRATION.**

- Treat for shock; see **SHOCK.**

SYMPTOMS

Vary from slight burning and mild swelling to acute pain and severe swelling. Can include: Nausea. Vomiting. Difficulty breathing. Dim or blurred vision. Weakness. Slurred speech. Sweating. Paralysis. Convulsions.

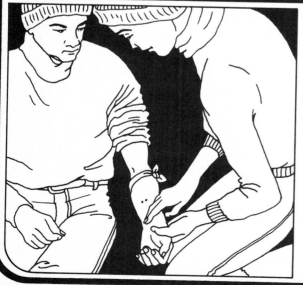

1 Apply a constricting band between the bite and the heart 2 to 4 inches above the puncture. **Do not** bind too tightly. Check the pulse below the wound; see **TAKING THE PULSE.** If you can't feel the pulse, loosen the band until it returns. The wound should ooze. Keep the affected part below heart level.

SNAKEBITE

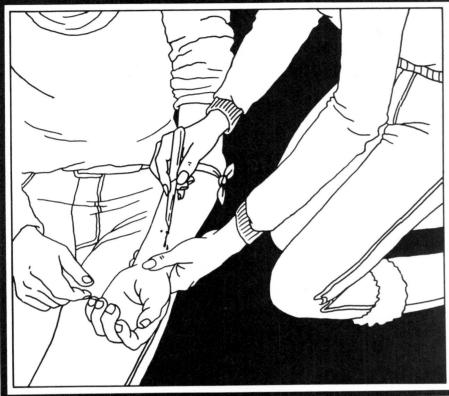

2 Clean the wound with alcohol or soap and water. Sterilize a knife or razor blade over an open flame, and make a **shallow (about ⅛ inch) vertical incision ½ inch long over each fang mark. Do not** cut deeply or crisscross. **Do not** make incisions on the head, neck or torso.

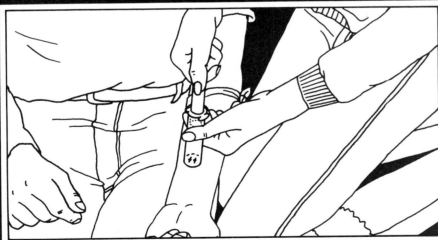

3 Draw the venom from the wound with a suction cup or with your mouth, if it is free of open sores. **Do not** swallow the venom. Continue suction for 30 minutes.

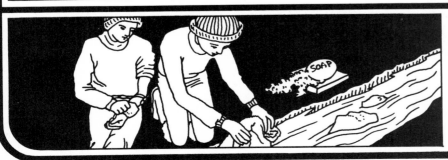

4 Wash thoroughly with soap and water. **Seek medical aid immediately.**

BLACK EYE

IMPORTANT

- Consult a doctor to determine if there is a more serious injury.

SYMPTOMS

Pain following a blow to the eye. Rapid swelling and dark discoloration of the eyelid or skin around the eye. Discoloration may last for 2 to 3 weeks.

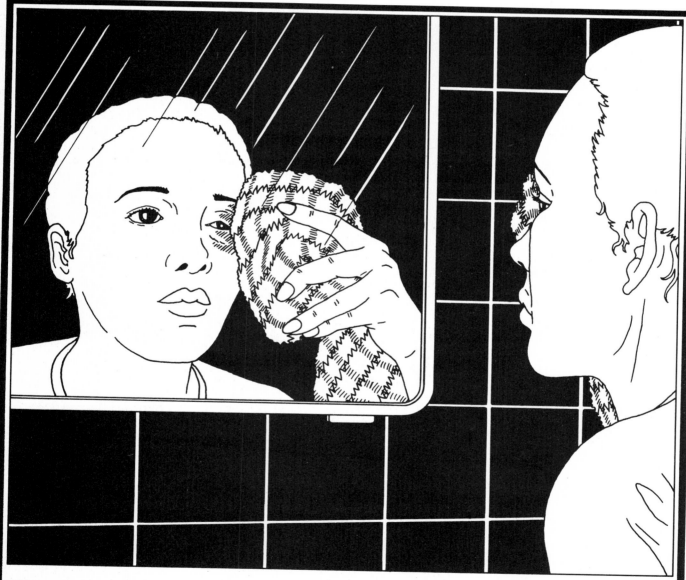

To minimize swelling, apply an ice bag covered with a towel to the affected area. If an ice bag isn't available, use ice cubes wrapped in a cloth. **Do not** place ice directly on the skin or eye.

DIRECT PRESSURE

IMPORTANT

- Seek medical aid for any serious bleeding.

- **Do not** apply direct pressure on breaks.

- Observe for shock; see **SHOCK.**

- **First try to control the bleeding by direct pressure; see below.**

- **If you cannot control the bleeding, use pressure points while continuing direct pressure; see BLEEDING: CUTS & WOUNDS (PRESSURE POINTS).**

- **If serious blood loss continues and becomes critical, apply a tourniquet as a last resort; see BLEEDING: CUTS & WOUNDS (TOURNIQUET).**

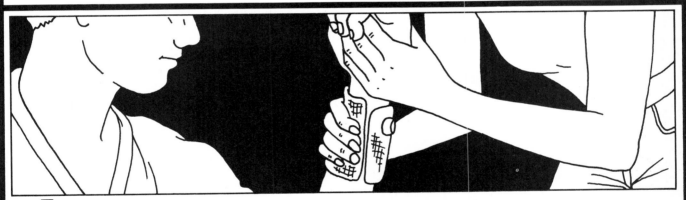

1 Press gauze or a clean cloth directly over the wound.

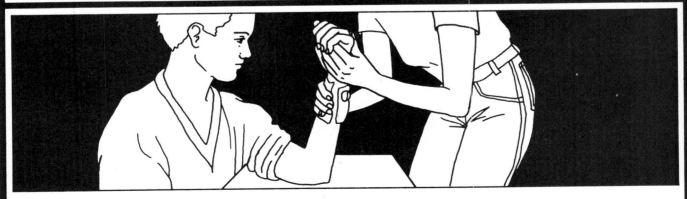

2 Elevate injured limbs higher than the heart unless there is evidence of fracture or it causes pain.

CONTINUED ON NEXT PAGE

DIRECT PRESSURE
CONTINUED

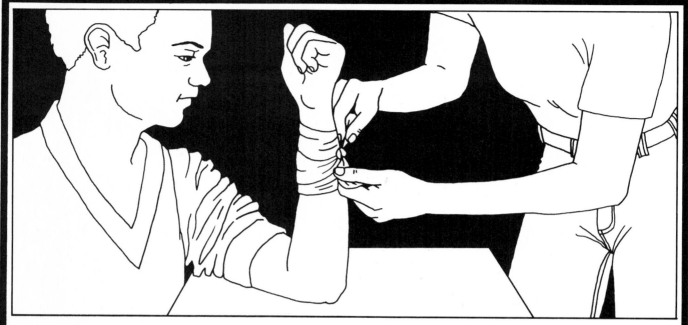

3 After bleeding is controlled, bandage firmly but not too tightly.

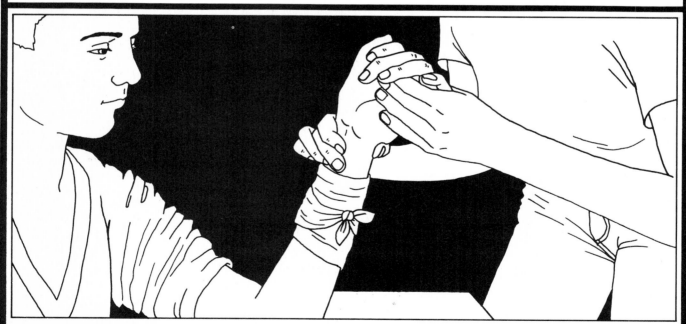

4 Check the pulse below the wound; see **TAKING THE PULSE.** If you can't feel the pulse, loosen the bandage until it returns, then treat for shock; see **SHOCK.**

PRESSURE POINTS

IMPORTANT

- **Seek medical aid for any serious bleeding.**
- Continue direct pressure.
- Observe for shock; see **SHOCK.**

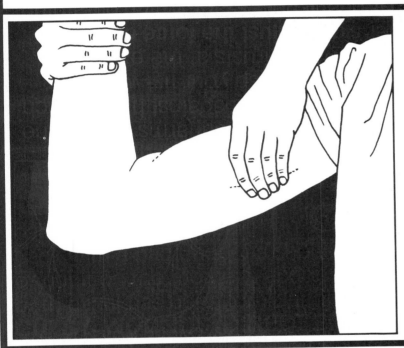

ARM

Elevate the injured arm higher than the heart unless there is evidence of fracture or it causes pain. Place your fingers on the inner side of the arm, pressing in the groove between the muscles. Keeping your thumb on the outside of the arm, press toward the bone.

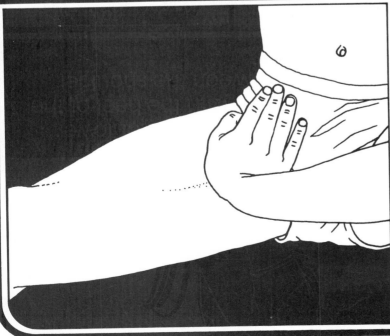

LEG

Elevate the injured leg higher than the heart unless there is evidence of fracture or it causes pain. Place the heel of your hand on the inner thigh at the midpoint of the crease of the groin. With your arm straight and your elbow locked, press against the bone.

TOURNIQUET

IMPORTANT

- **Seek medical aid immediately.**

- **Use of a tourniquet may necessitate later amputation of the limb. Do not use except in a critical emergency where all other methods fail to control serious bleeding. First try direct pressure and pressure points; see BLEEDING: CUTS & WOUNDS (DIRECT PRESSURE) and BLEEDING: CUTS & WOUNDS (PRESSURE POINTS).**

- **The tourniquet band must be at least 2 inches wide.**

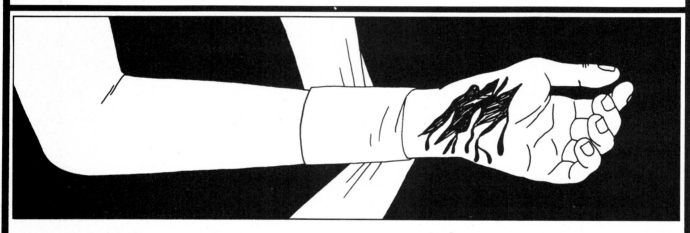

1 Place the tourniquet band over the artery to be compressed, slightly **above** the wound (about ½ inch). If a joint intervenes, position the band above the joint.

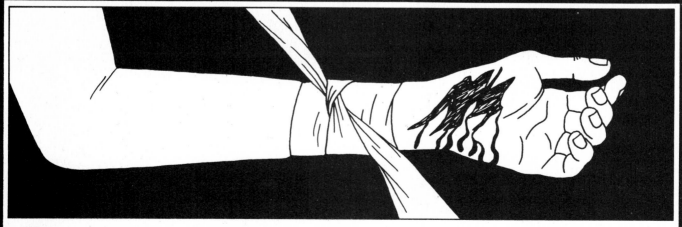

2 Wrap the band tightly around the limb twice, and tie a half-knot.

TOURNIQUET

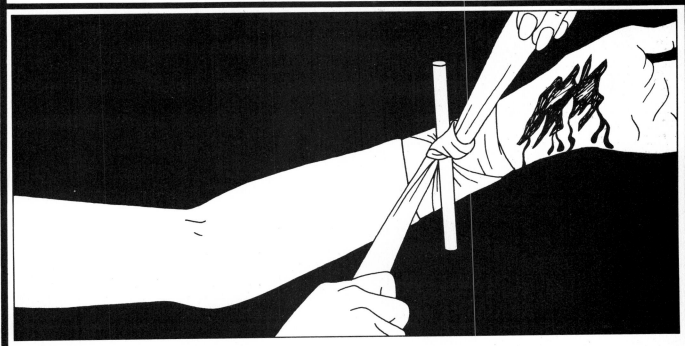

3 Place a short, strong stick on the band, and complete the knot on the top of the stick.

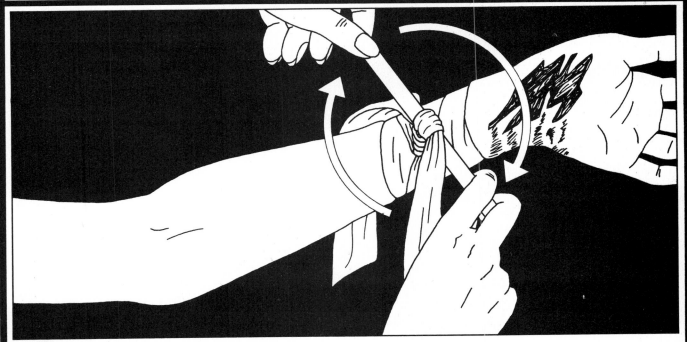

4 Twist the stick until the bleeding stops.

CONTINUED ON NEXT PAGE

TOURNIQUET
CONTINUED

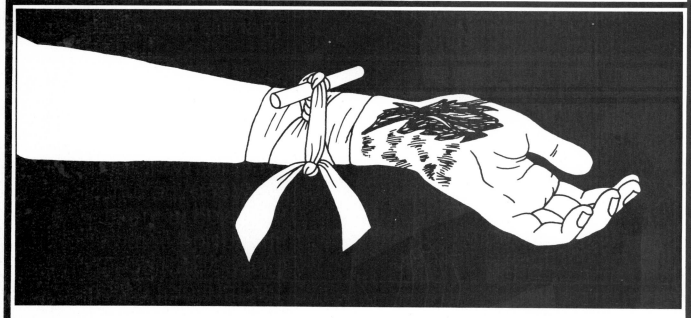

5 Secure the stick in place. **Do not** loosen unless a doctor so advises.

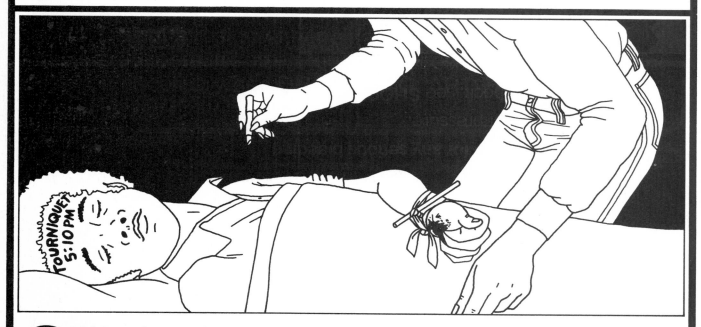

6 Write down the exact time the tourniquet was applied. Attach it as a note to the person's clothing or write it on his forehead with lipstick, etc. Treat for shock; see **SHOCK.** Get to a hospital immediately. **Do not** cover tourniquet.

AMPUTATIONS

IMPORTANT

- **Stay calm and act quickly.** Bleeding must be stopped as soon as possible.

- **Seek medical aid immediately.**

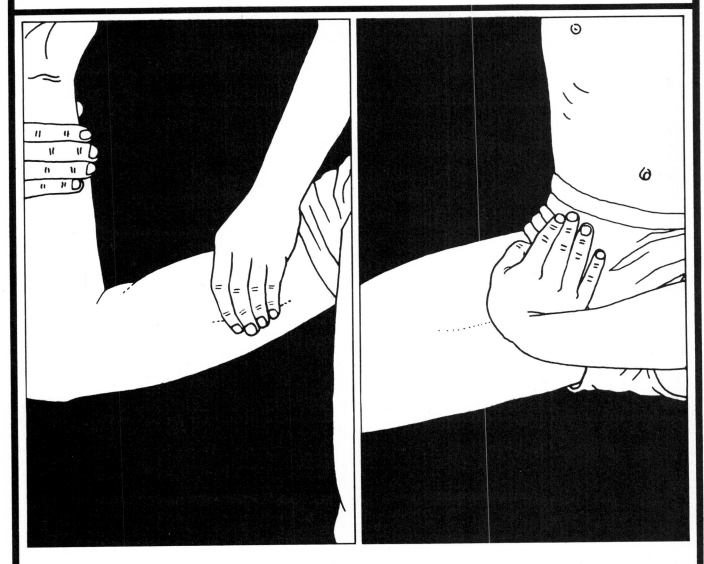

1 Control the bleeding through direct pressure and pressure points; see **BLEEDING: CUTS & WOUNDS (DIRECT PRESSURE)** and **BLEEDING: CUTS & WOUNDS (PRESSURE POINTS).** As a last resort, a tourniquet may be necessary; see **BLEEDING: CUTS & WOUNDS (TOURNIQUET).**

CONTINUED ON NEXT PAGE

AMPUTATIONS
CONTINUED

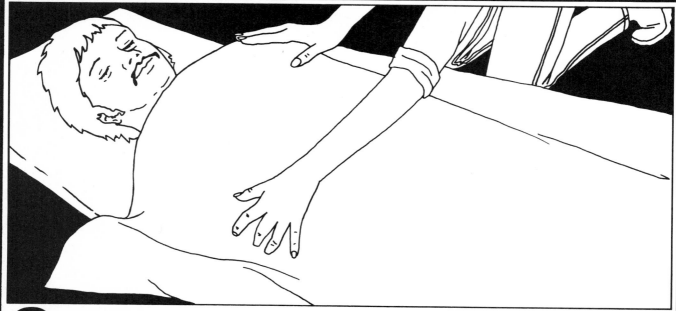

2 Treat for shock; see **SHOCK.**

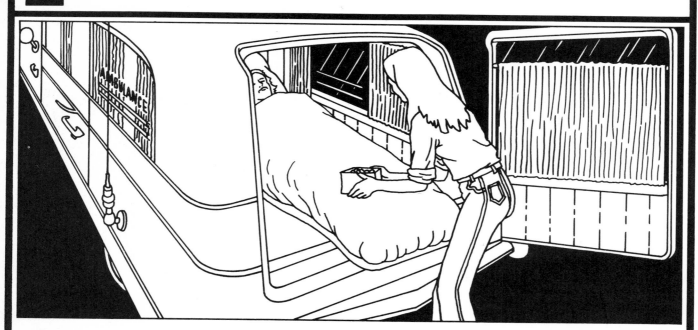

3 Wrap severed parts in a dry, clean dressing, then place in a plastic bag and keep cool. Transport to the hospital with the person. If an ambulance isn't available, see **TRANSPORTING THE INJURED.**

BLEEDING: CUTS & WOUNDS

FISHHOOKS

IMPORTANT

- **Do not** attempt to remove a fishhook from the face. **Seek medical aid immediately.**

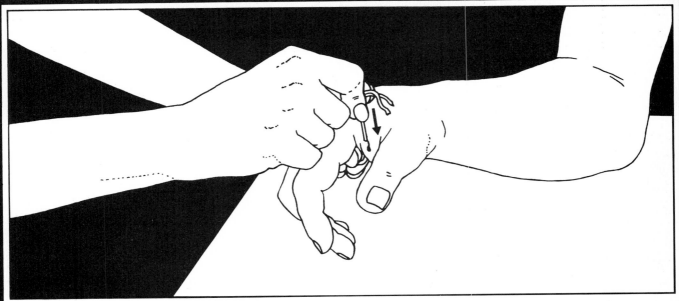

1 Push the shank through the skin until the point appears.

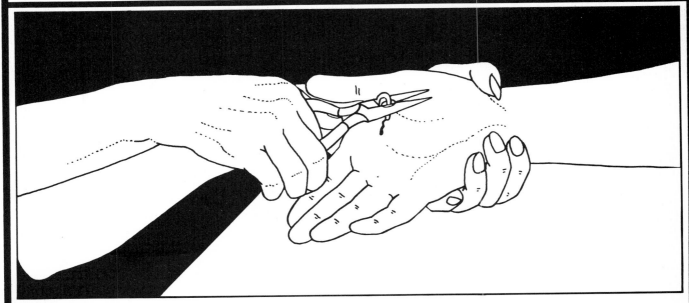

2 Cut off the barbed end with clippers or pliers.

CONTINUED ON NEXT PAGE

FISHHOOKS
CONTINUED

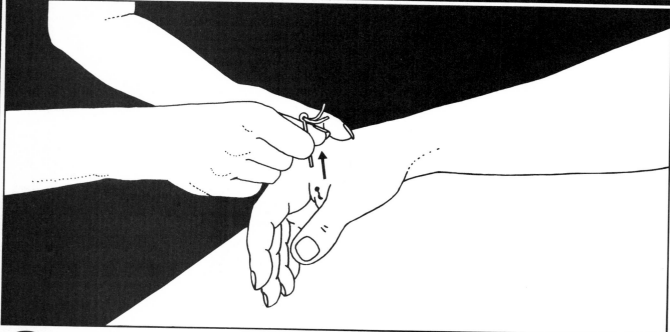

3 Remove the shank from the wound.

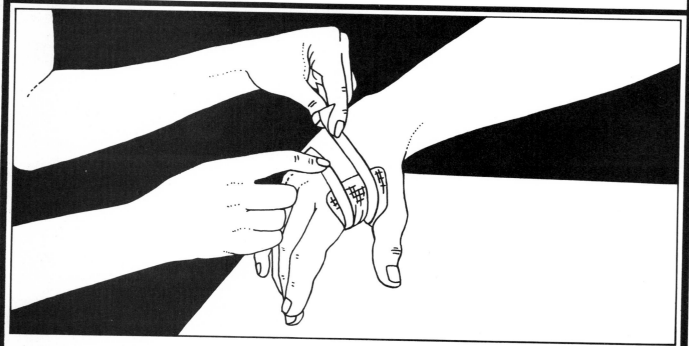

4 Wash the wound with soap and water. Cover with gauze or a clean cloth. **Consult your doctor.**

IMPALED OBJECTS

IMPORTANT

- **Call for an ambulance or get to the hospital immediately.**
  If necessary, see **TRANSPORTING THE INJURED.**

- **Do not** move the person off an impaling object unless his life is in imminent danger. If you must, remove him as gently as possible, tend to his wounds immediately, and treat for shock; see **SHOCK.**

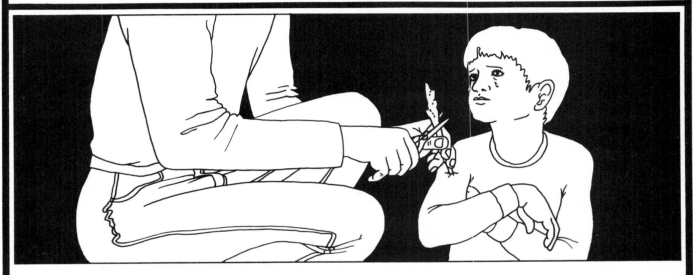

1 If possible, cut off the impaled object several inches from the wound without moving or removing it.

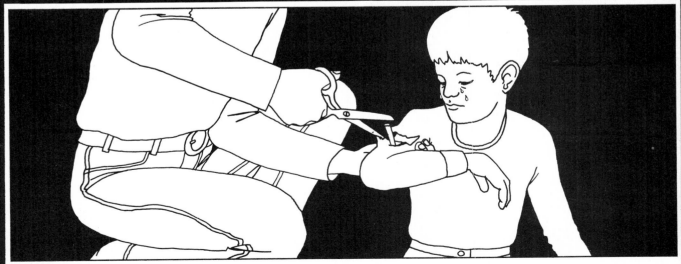

2 Carefully cut away the clothing from around the wound.

CONTINUED ON NEXT PAGE

IMPALED OBJECTS
CONTINUED

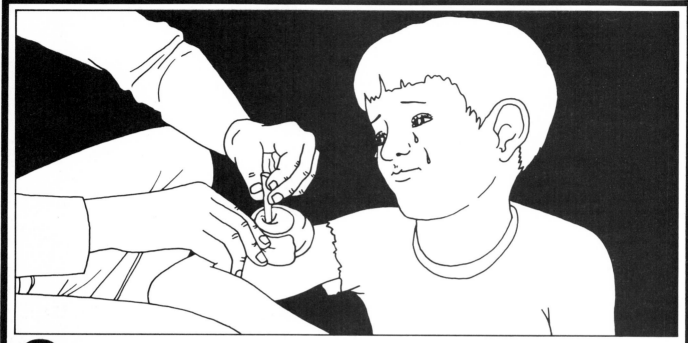

3 Immobilize the object by placing bulky dressings around it.

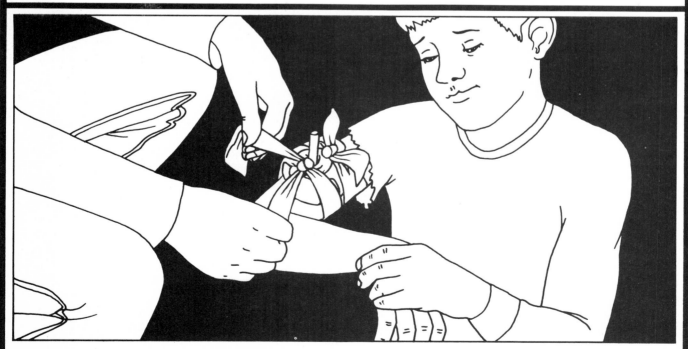

4 Secure the dressings in place with bandages. Treat for shock; see **SHOCK.**

INTERNAL BLEEDING

IMPORTANT

- To be suspected if the person has had a sharp blow or crushing injury to the abdomen, chest or torso.

- **Seek medical aid immediately.**

- **Do not** give the person anything to drink.

SYMPTOMS

Stomach: Vomit is bright red, dark red or the color and size of large coffee grounds.

Intestines: Excrement contains dark tar-like material or bright red blood.

Chest and Lungs: Bright red foamy blood is coughed up.

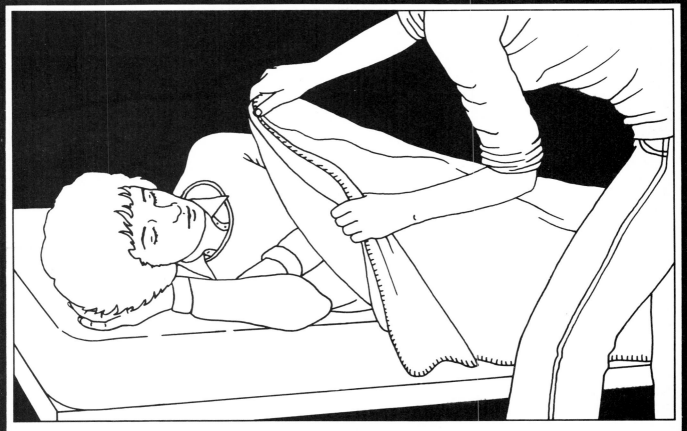

1 Keep the person lying down and covered lightly. Turn the head to one side to keep the air passage clear.

CONTINUED ON NEXT PAGE

INTERNAL BLEEDING
CONTINUED

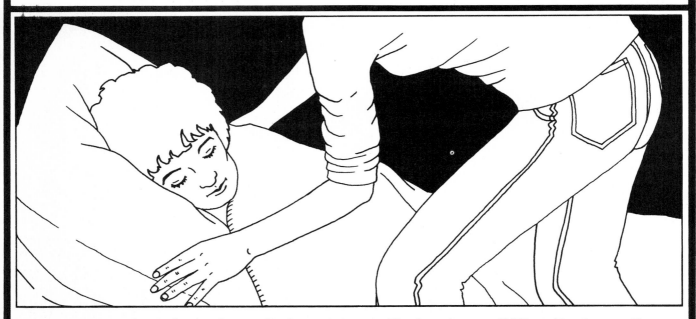

2 Raise her head and shoulders if she has difficulty breathing. If necessary, see **BREATHING: ARTIFICIAL RESPIRATION.**

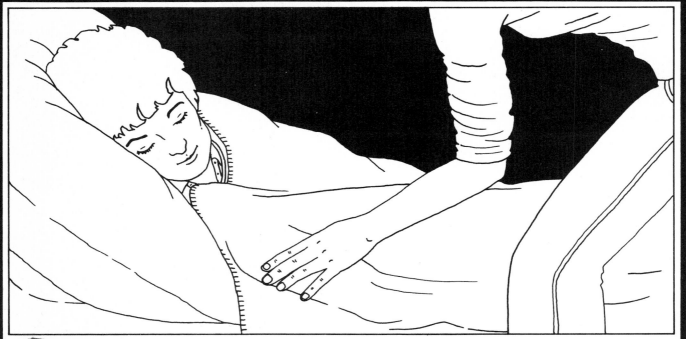

3 Treat for shock; see **SHOCK.**

BLISTERS

IMPORTANT

- **Seek medical aid** if blisters are large, affect deep tissues of the hands or soles of the feet, cover a large portion of the body or become infected.

- **Do not** break or open blisters caused by burns, frostbite or irritation from insect bites, poison ivy or heat rash.

SYMPTOMS

A well-defined cushion-like raised area filled with clear fluid. May be uncomfortable or painful, particularly if broken.

IF THE BLISTER IS UNBROKEN

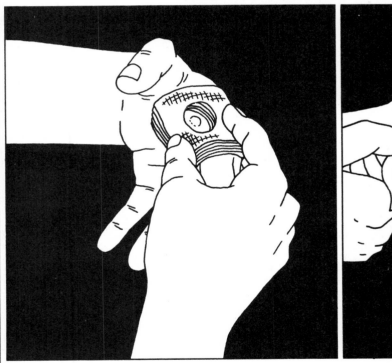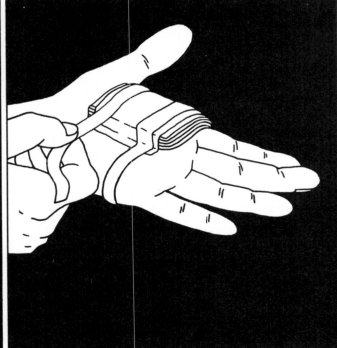

Try to protect the blister from breaking by improvising a shield. Cut a hole in the center of several gauze pads slightly larger than the affected area. Place the hole in each pad over the blister, taking care not to touch the blister. Add sufficient layers to protect the blister from contact, then cover the opening with a pad fastened loosely in place with adhesive tape. If possible, **do not** use the affected area.

BLISTERS

IF YOU CANNOT PREVENT THE BLISTER FROM BREAKING

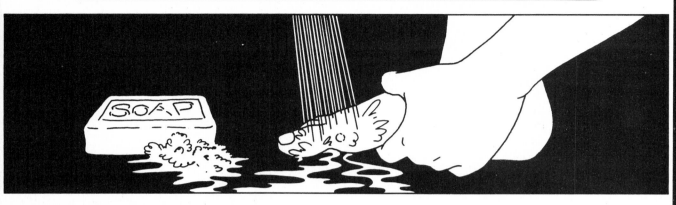

1 Gently wash the affected area thoroughly with soap and water.

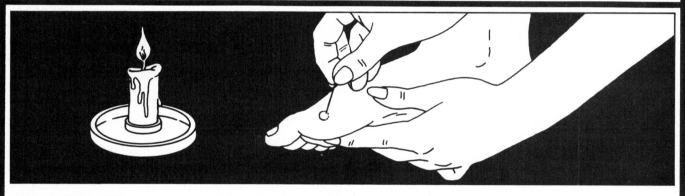

2 Sterilize a needle by holding it over an open flame or soaking it in rubbing alcohol, then carefully puncture the edge of the blister to allow fluids to drain out.

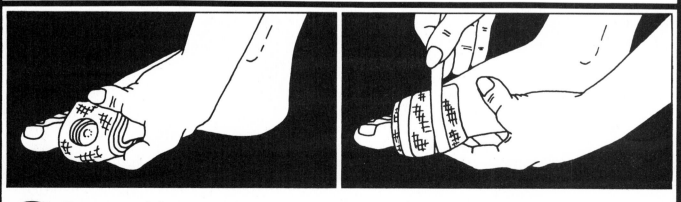

3 Cover with a sterile gauze pad or clean cloth held in place with adhesive tape.

BLISTERS

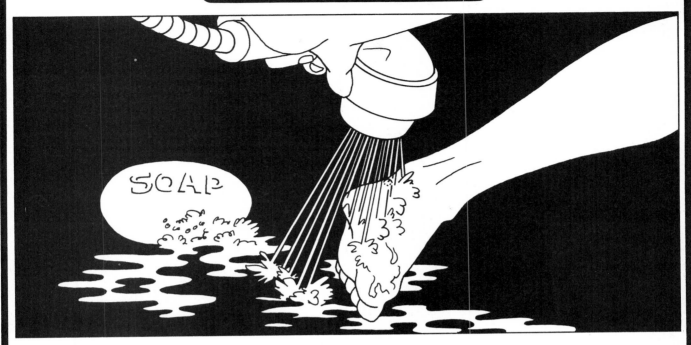

1 Gently wash the affected area thoroughly with soap and water.

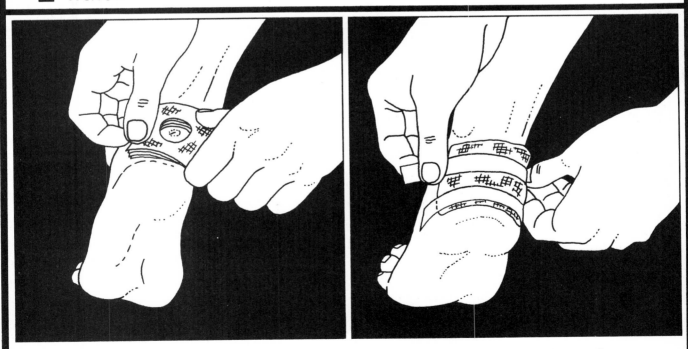

2 Improvise a shield with gauze pads; see procedure for unbroken blister.

BOILS & CARBUNCLES

IMPORTANT

- **Seek medical aid,** particularly if the central area of the face, under-arm or groin is affected or if the boils spread, form clusters (carbuncles) or become chronic.

- **Do not** puncture or squeeze boils.

SYMPTOMS

Caused by inflamed and infected hair follicles. Usually take 3 to 5 days to develop. Often affect the skin of the face, neck, chest or buttocks. Itching. Redness. Tenderness or acute pain. Possible throbbing. May come to a head, open and drain a mixture of pus and blood. **In severe cases:** May spread and form clusters. Chills. Fever.

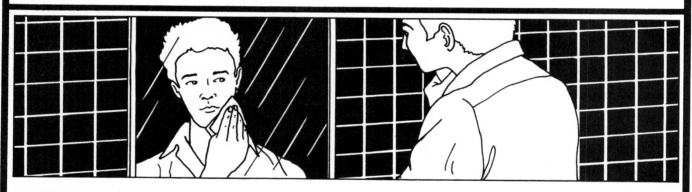

1 Apply hot wet compresses to affected area for 10 minutes, 3 to 4 times a day. Between compresses, avoid pressure or friction by covering the affected area with a gauze pad or clean cloth loosely fastened in place with adhesive tape. Continue until the boil comes to a head, opens by itself and begins to drain.

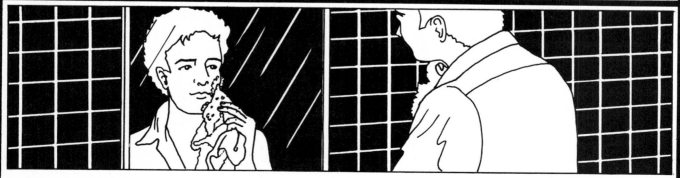

2 After the boil opens, use soap and water to help keep the area clean and free of debris.

BOILS & CARBUNCLES

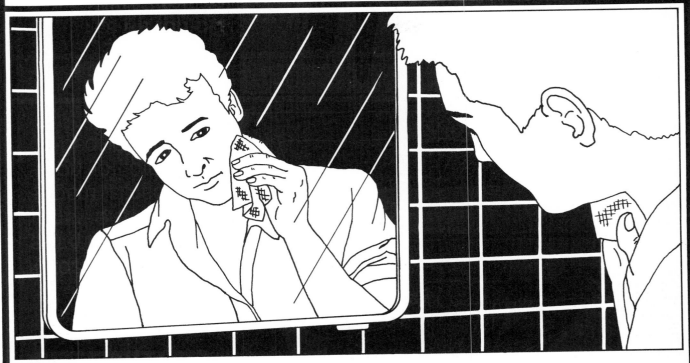

3 Gently blot dry with sterile gauze or clean cloth.

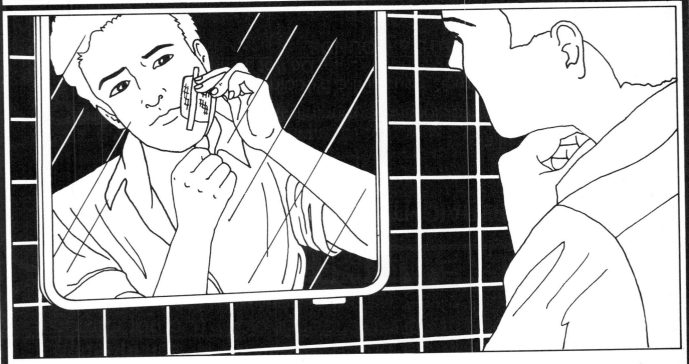

4 Cover with a clean, nonadhering dressing or cloth. Hold the dressing in place with adhesive tape.

COLLARBONE, SHOULDER & BENT ELBOW

IMPORTANT

- **Seek medical aid.**

- **Do not** try to reset dislocations yourself. Treat the same as fractures.

- If any bones protrude, control the bleeding and cover the wound with a large clean dressing or cloth. **Do not** clean the wound. See **BLEEDING: CUTS & WOUNDS.**

- Treat for shock; see **SHOCK.**

COLLARBONE & SHOULDER

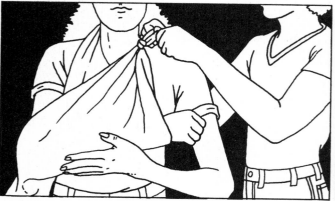 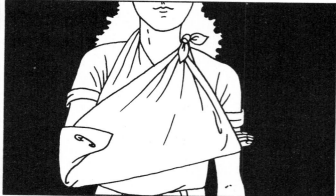

1 Make a sling to support the weight of the arm, with the hand 4 to 5 inches above the elbow.

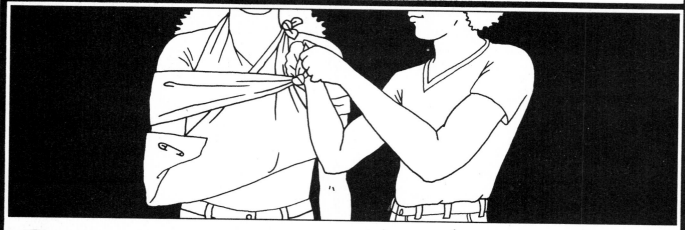

2 Immobilize the arm by tying a band over the sling and around the body.

COLLARBONE, SHOULDER & BENT ELBOW

BENT ELBOW

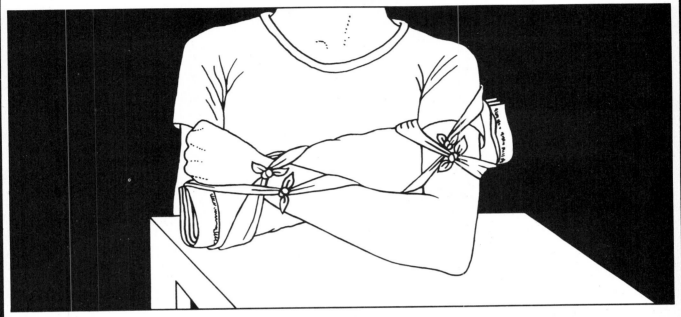

1 Immobilize in the position found with a padded splint. Use boards, magazines, etc. for rigidity; cloth for padding.

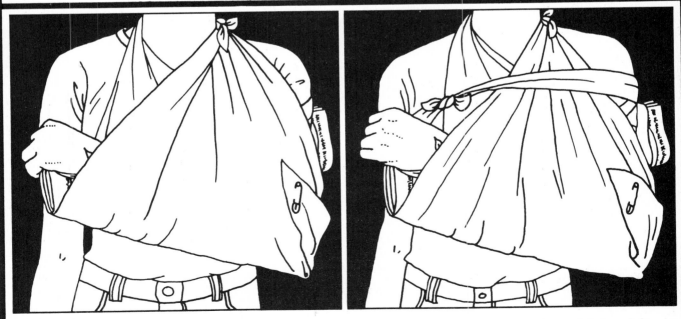

2 Make a sling to support the weight of the arm, and bind it to the body. Be sure the fingers are above elbow level.

STRAIGHT ELBOW & FINGER

IMPORTANT

- **Seek medical aid.**

- **Do not** try to reset dislocations yourself. Treat the same as fractures.

- If any bones protrude, control the bleeding and cover the wound with a large clean dressing or cloth. **Do not** clean the wound. See **BLEEDING: CUTS & WOUNDS.**

- Treat for shock; see **SHOCK.**

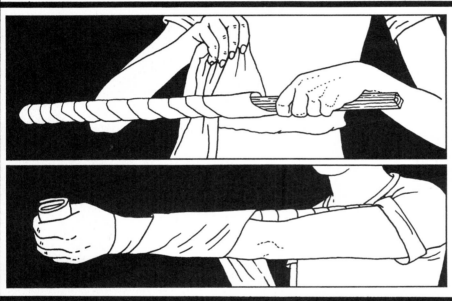

STRAIGHT ELBOW

Immobilize the elbow in position with a padded splint extending from the armpit to the hand. Use boards, magazines, etc. for rigidity; cloth for padding.

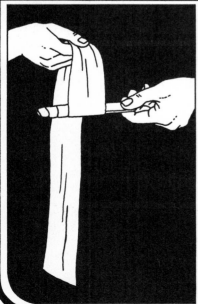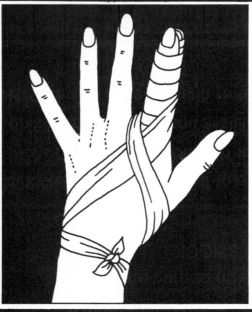

FINGER

Do not try to straighten the finger. Immobilize it in position with a padded splint made from a tongue depressor or the like. Bind the splint to the finger with cloth or tape.

ARM, WRIST & HAND

IMPORTANT

- **Seek medical aid.**

- **Do not** try to reset dislocations yourself. Treat the same as fractures.

- If any bones protrude, control the bleeding and cover the wound with a large clean dressing or cloth. **Do not** clean the wound. See **BLEEDING: CUTS & WOUNDS.**

- Treat for shock; see **SHOCK.**

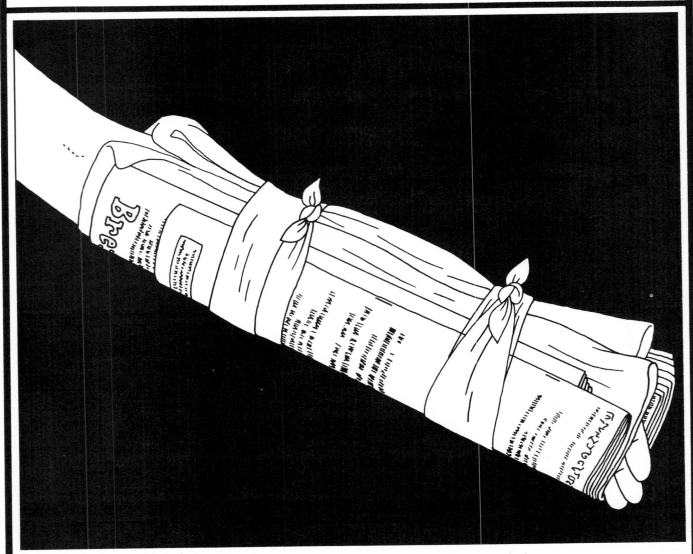

1 Immobilize with a padded splint. Use boards, magazines, etc. for rigidity; cloth for padding. **Do not** tie too tightly.

CONTINUED ON NEXT PAGE

ARM, WRIST & HAND
CONTINUED

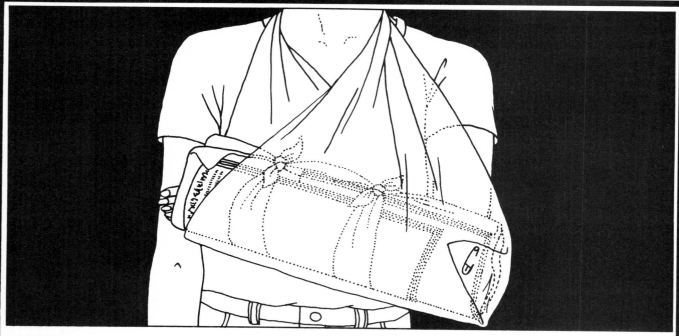

2 Make a sling to support the weight of the arm. Be sure the fingers are above elbow level.

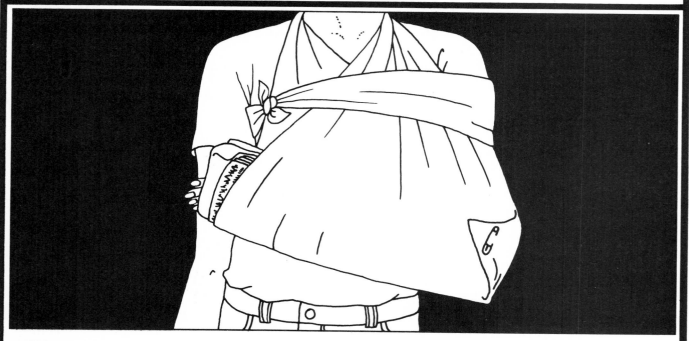

3 For a broken arm, immobilize the shoulder and elbow by binding the arm to the body.

PELVIS & HIP

IMPORTANT

- **Seek medical aid.**
- **Do not** try to reset dislocations yourself. Treat the same as fractures.
- Treat for shock; see **SHOCK.**

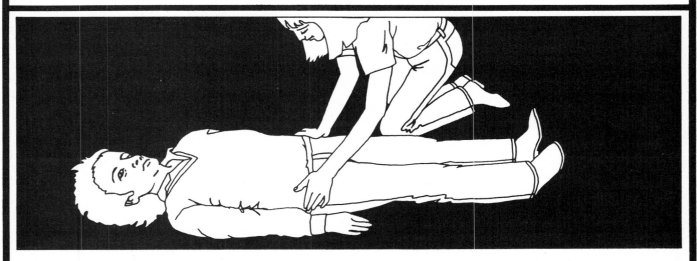

1 Check for fracture by gently feeling the bones in the pelvic and hip areas. Note where it hurts the person when you touch him.

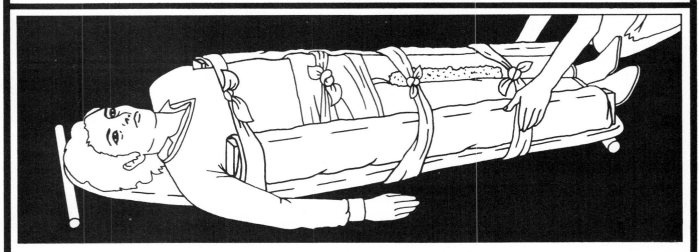

2 To immobilize the person, place thick padding between his thighs, then tie him down on a board, door, etc. with bandages, belts or the like.

BREAKS: FRACTURES & DISLOCATIONS

KNEE, LEG & ANKLE

IMPORTANT

- **Seek medical aid.**
- **Do not** try to reset dislocations yourself. Treat the same as fractures.
- Treat for shock; see **SHOCK**.

KNEE

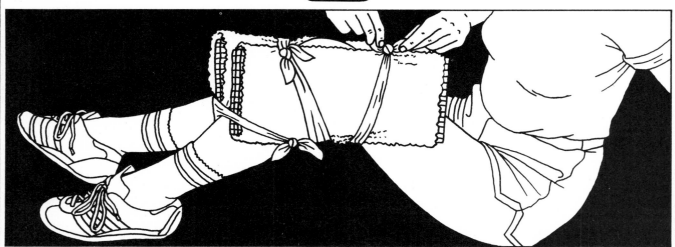

1A Immobilize in the position found with a padded splint. Use boards, magazines, etc. for rigidity; cloth for padding.

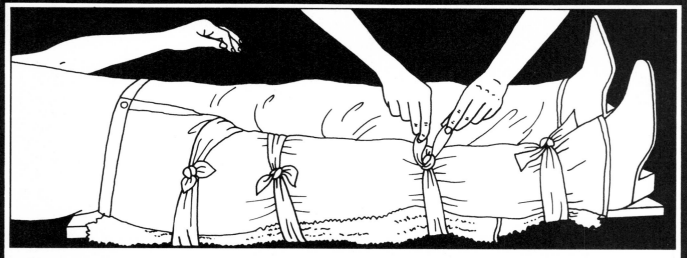

1B For a straight knee, extend the splint from the buttock to the heel.

BREAKS: FRACTURES & DISLOCATIONS

KNEE, LEG & ANKLE

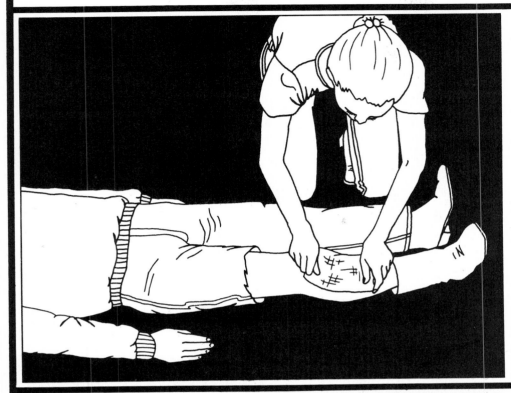

LEG & ANKLE

1 If any bones protrude, control the bleeding and cover with a large clean dressing or cloth. **Do not** clean the wound. See **BLEEDING: CUTS & WOUNDS.**

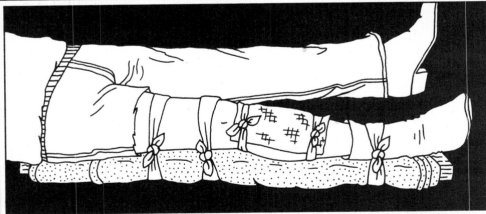

2A Immobilize with a padded splint. Use boards, magazines, etc. for rigidity; cloth or a pillow for padding.

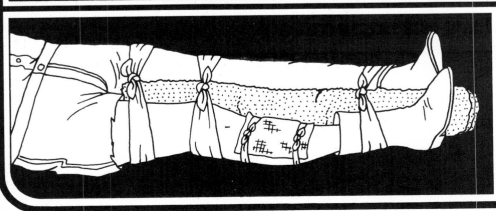

2B If unable to improvise a splint, place padding between the legs and tie them together.

FOOT & TOE

IMPORTANT

- **Seek medical aid.**

- **Do not** try to reset dislocations yourself. Treat the same as fractures.

- If any bones protrude, control the bleeding and cover the wound with a large clean dressing or cloth. **Do not** clean the wound. See **BLEEDING: CUTS & WOUNDS.**

- Treat for shock; see **SHOCK.**

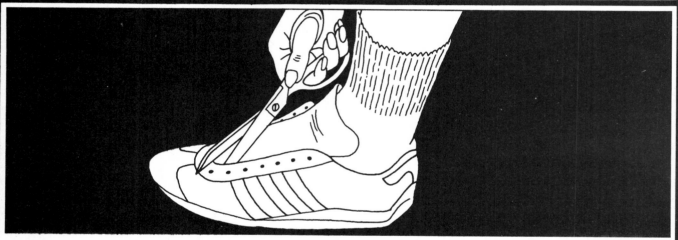

1 Try to remove or cut away the shoe.

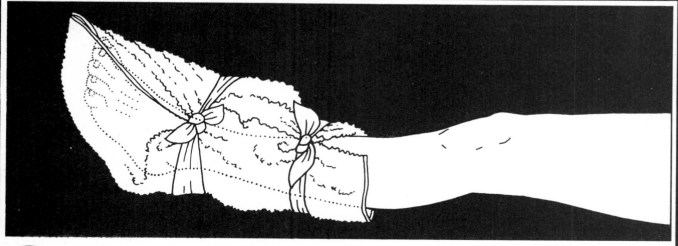

2 Immobilize with a padded splint made from a blanket, pillow, etc. Tie it snugly but not too tightly.

BREATHING: ARTIFICIAL RESPIRATION

INFANT & SMALL CHILD

IMPORTANT

- **Seek medical aid as quickly as possible.**

- **Do not** tip back the head if there is a neck or back injury. To open the air passage, gently pull open the jaw without moving the head.

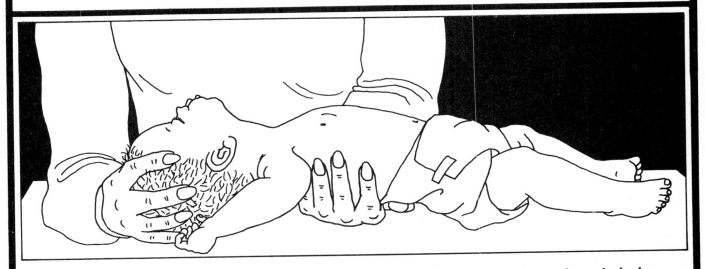

1 Place the child on his back. If there is no neck or back injury, open the air passage by gently tipping back his head. If necessary, clear out his mouth with your fingers or a cloth.

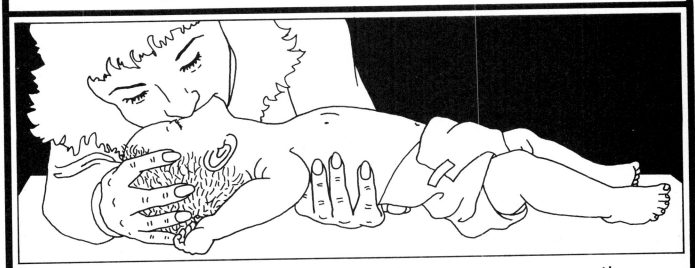

2 **If breathing does not resume,** place your open mouth over the child's nose and mouth, forming an airtight seal. Give 4 quick gentle breaths.

CONTINUED ON NEXT PAGE

INFANT & SMALL CHILD
CONTINUED

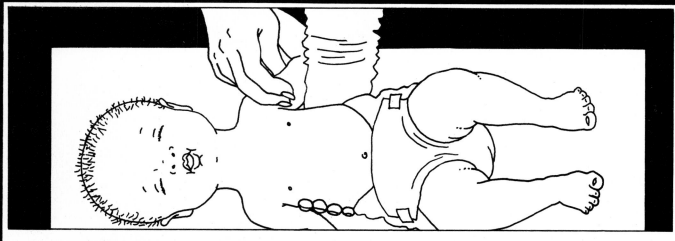

3A **If breathing still has not resumed,** check the pulse on the inside of the upper arm. If you cannot feel it, see **HEART FAILURE.**

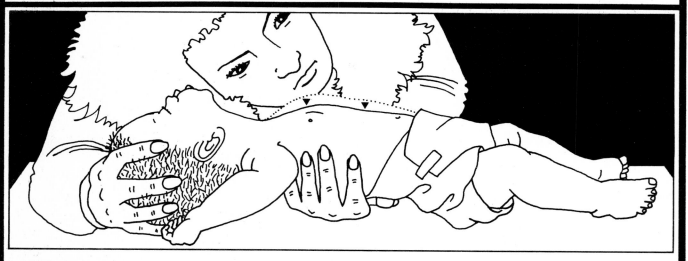

3B **If there is a pulse,** then give the child a new breath every 3 seconds, 20 per minute, using short gentle puffs of air. Remove your mouth between breaths and look and listen for the air leaving his lungs. If the entry or return of air seems blocked or the chest does not move, see **CHOKING,** then resume artificial respiration at Step 1. Continue until the child breathes spontaneously or professional help arrives. Treat for shock; see **SHOCK.**

OLDER CHILD & ADULT

(IMPORTANT)

- **Seek medical aid as quickly as possible.**

- **Do not** tip back the head if there is a neck or back injury. To open the air passage, gently pull open the jaw without moving the head.

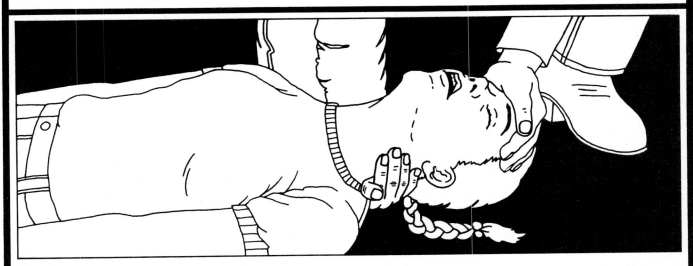

1 Place the person on her back. If there is no neck or back injury, open the air passage by gently tipping back her head. If necessary, clear out her mouth with your fingers or a cloth.

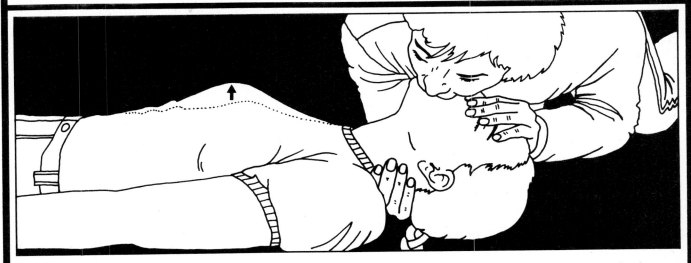

2 **If breathing does not resume,** open her jaws and pinch her nose closed. Place your mouth over her mouth, forming an airtight seal. Give 4 quick gentle breaths.

CONTINUED ON NEXT PAGE

OLDER CHILD & ADULT
CONTINUED

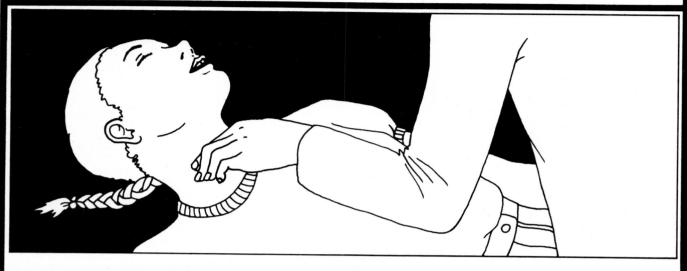

3A **If breathing still has not resumed,** check the pulse at the large artery in the neck. If you cannot feel it, see **HEART FAILURE.**

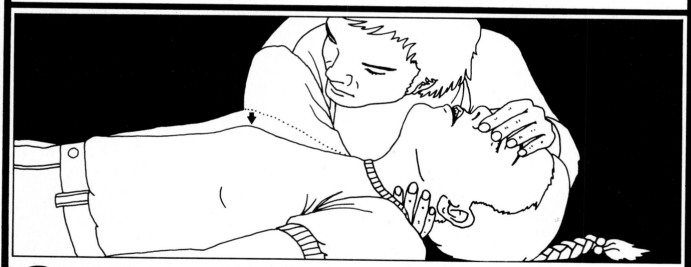

3B **If there is a pulse,** then give the person a new breath every 5 seconds, 12 per minute. Remove your mouth between breaths and look and listen for the air leaving her lungs. If the entry or return of air seems blocked or the chest does not move, see **CHOKING,** then resume artificial respiration at Step 1. Continue until the person breathes spontaneously or professional help arrives. Treat for shock; see **SHOCK.**

IMPORTANT

• Seek medical aid as soon as possible.

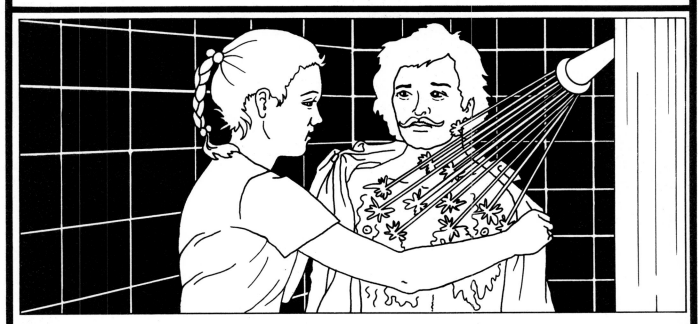

1A Place the person under a heavy, cool shower immediately. Remove all contamined clothing. Keep him there at least 5 minutes, until all traces of the chemical have washed away.

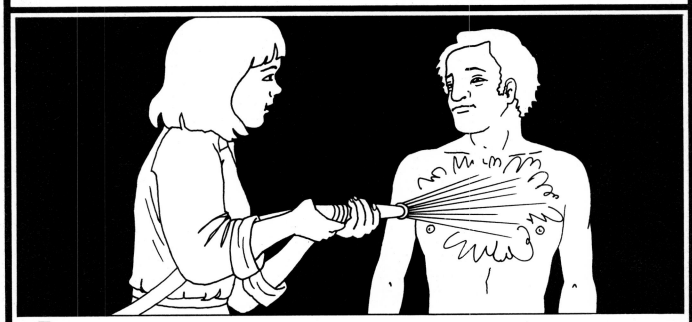

1B If a shower is not available, use a hose.

CONTINUED ON NEXT PAGE

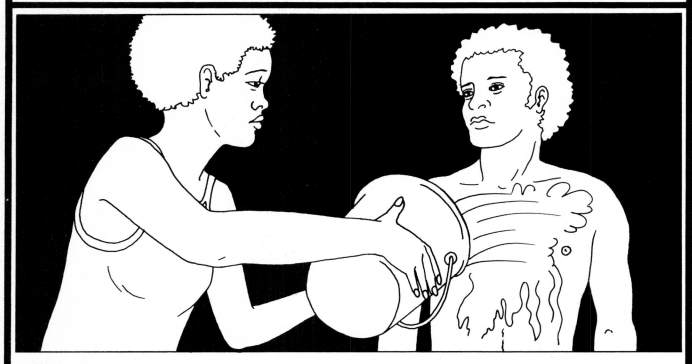

1c If a hose isn't available, keep pouring cool water over the burn.

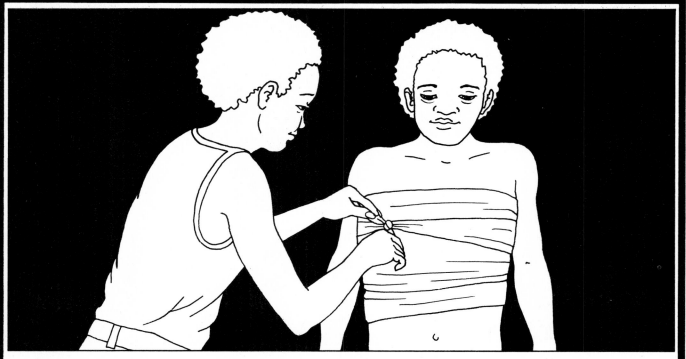

2 Cover with a clean, nonadhering dressing or cloth. Treat for shock; see **SHOCK.**

1st & 2nd DEGREE

IMPORTANT

- **Do not** remove shreds of tissue or break blisters.

- **Do not** use antiseptic sprays, ointments or home remedies.

- **Do not** put pressure on burned areas.

- Treat for shock; see **SHOCK.**

- **Seek medical aid.**

Determine the degree of the burn and treat accordingly:

- **First Degree: Red or discolored skin. See below.**

- **Second Degree: Blisters and red or mottled skin. See below.**

- **Third Degree: White or charred skin.** See **BURNS: HEAT (3rd DEGREE).**

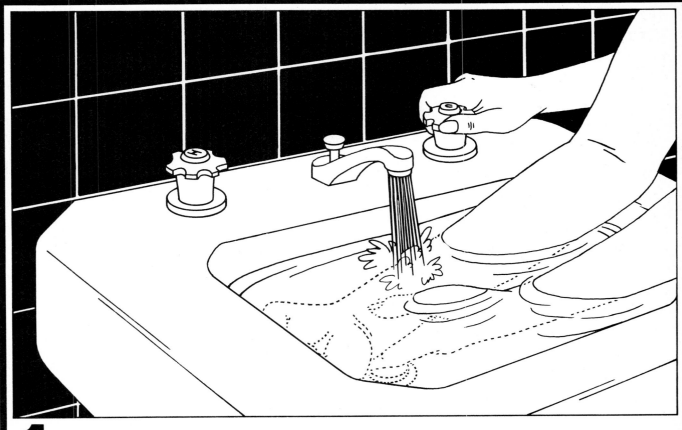

1A Immerse in cold (**not ice**) water until pain subsides.

CONTINUED ON NEXT PAGE

1st & 2nd DEGREE
CONTINUED

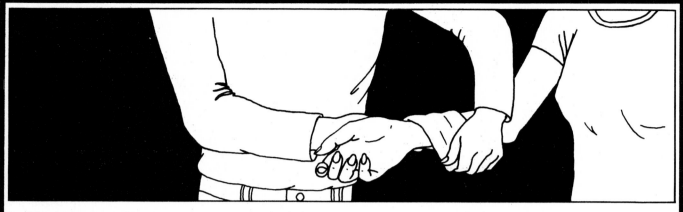

1B Or lightly apply cold clean compresses that have been wrung out in cold water.

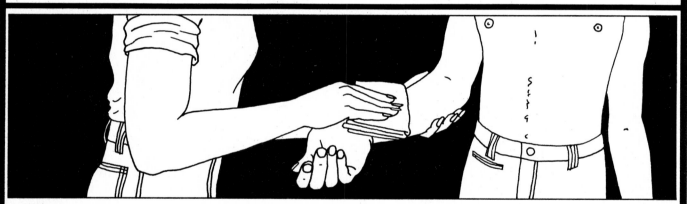

2 Gently blot dry with sterile gauze or a clean cloth.

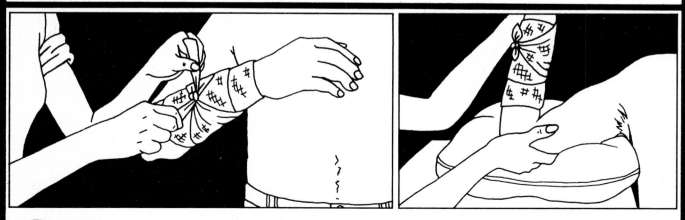

3 Cover loosely with a dry clean dressing. Elevate burned arms or legs higher than the heart.

3rd DEGREE

(IMPORTANT)

- **Call for an ambulance or doctor immediately.**

- **Do not** apply antiseptic sprays, ointments or home remedies.

- **Do not** apply ice to large burns or immerse them in water.

- **Do not** remove adhered particles of clothing.

- **Do not** remove shreds of tissue or break blisters.

- **Do not** use absorbent cotton.

- **If the person is unconscious or vomiting, do not** give him anything to drink.

- **Do not** give the person anything alcoholic to drink.

- Treat for shock; see **SHOCK.**

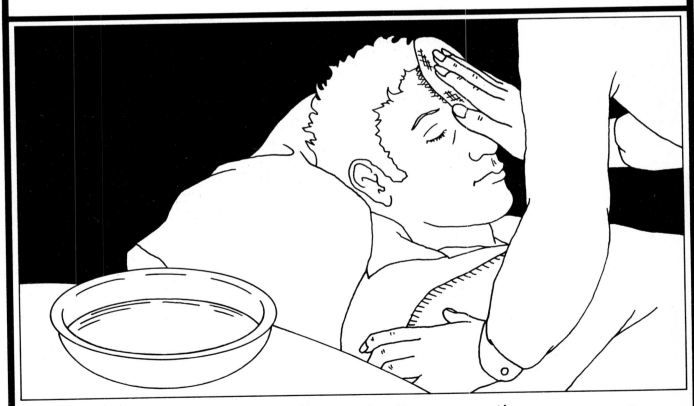

1A If the face has been burned, sit or prop the person up and apply a cold compress. Watch breathing closely. If necessary, see **BREATHING: ARTIFICIAL RESPIRATION.**

CONTINUED ON NEXT PAGE

3rd DEGREE
CONTINUED

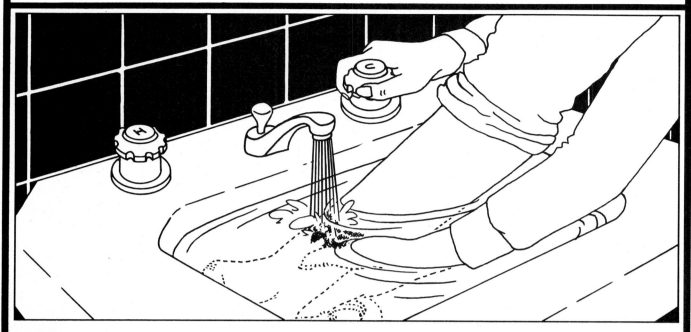

1B Immerse small localized burns in cold (**not ice**) water until pain subsides.

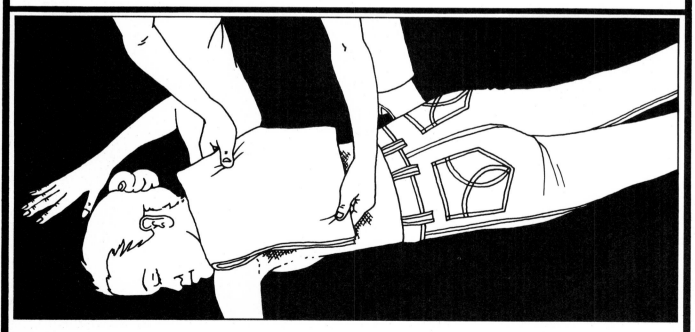

1C Lightly cover larger burned areas with a nonadhering dressing or a dry clean sheet or cloth. (**Do not** immerse them in cold water or cover them with ice.)

3rd DEGREE

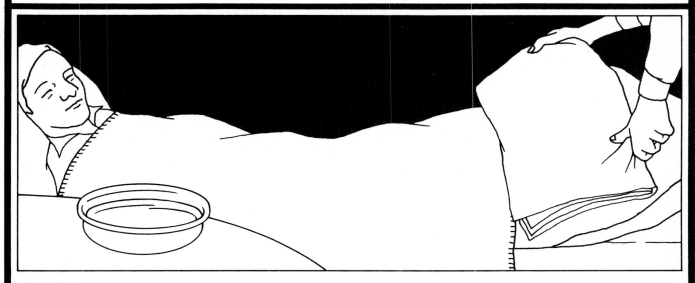

2 Elevate burned arms or legs higher than the heart and apply a cold compress.

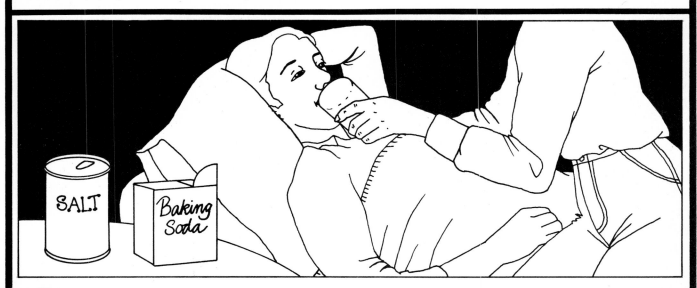

3 If you cannot obtain professional medical care for an hour or more and the person is conscious and not vomiting, have him sip about 4 ounces of water (2 ounces for a child over 1 year of age, 1 ounce for an infant) containing salt and baking soda (1 level teaspoon salt and ½ level teaspoon baking soda **per quart** of lukewarm water). Discontinue liquid if the person vomits. **Do not** give an unconscious person anything to drink.

CHEST INJURIES

CRUSHED CHEST

IMPORTANT

- **Seek medical aid immediately.**
- Treat for shock; see **SHOCK.**

SYMPTOMS

Many broken ribs. The chest may collapse rather than expand when the person tries to inhale.

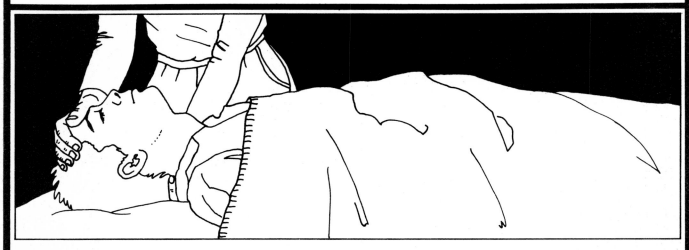

1 Open the person's air passage by gently tipping back his head.

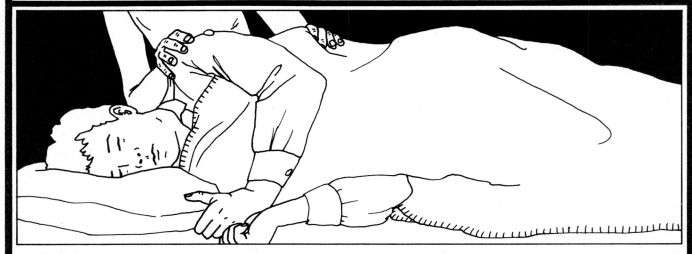

2A If the injury is only on one side, turn the injured side down if possible, and try to make the person comfortable.

CHEST INJURIES

CRUSHED CHEST

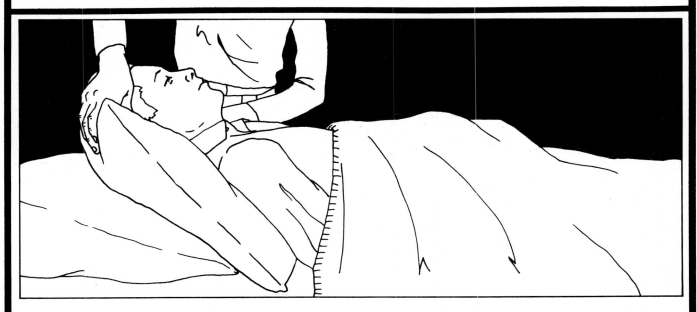

2B If the injury is in the center of the chest or on both sides or if the person has trouble breathing, prop him up in a comfortable position.

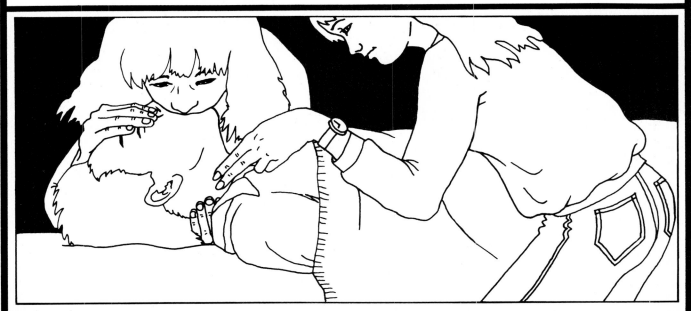

3 If necessary, begin rescue breathing immediately; see **BREATHING: ARTIFICIAL RESPIRATION.** Watch his pulse closely; see **TAKING THE PULSE.** If it stops, treat for heart failure immediately; see **HEART FAILURE.**

CHEST INJURIES

OPEN CHEST WOUNDS

IMPORTANT

• **Seek medical aid immediately.**

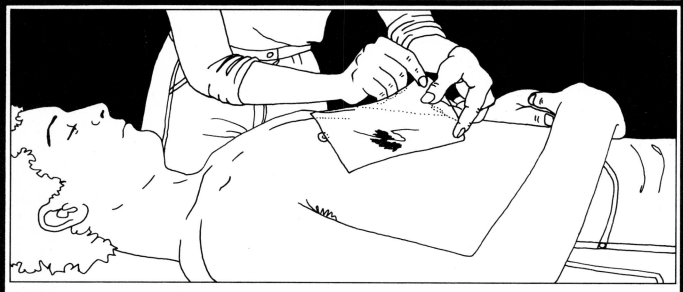

1 Seal the wound immediately with a nonporous dressing — plastic tape, aluminum foil, etc.

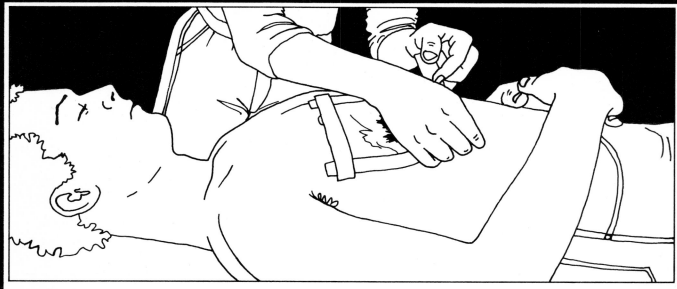

2 Tape the seal in place. If tape is not available, bind the seal with a wide bandage, belt or the like. Be careful not to restrict breathing.

CHEST INJURIES

OPEN CHEST WOUNDS

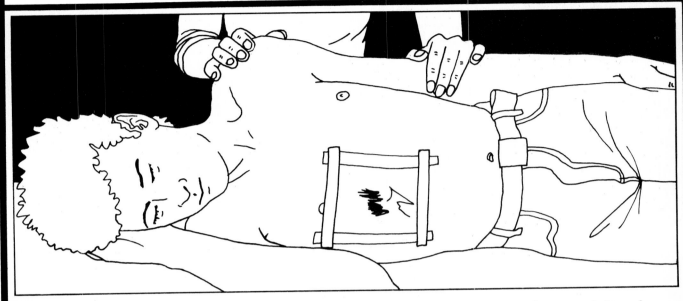

3 Turn the person onto the injured side to help keep his air passage open. Treat for shock; see **SHOCK**.

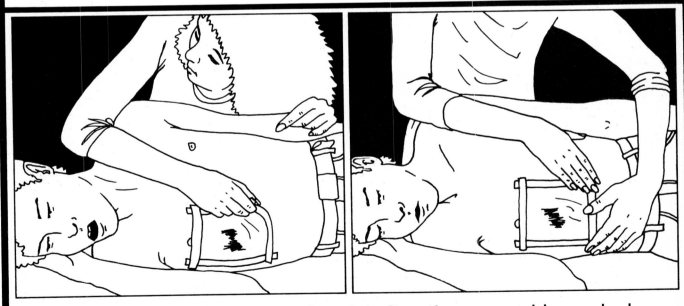

4 If the person worsens shortly after the wound is sealed, his lung may have collapsed, in which case remove the seal immediately while the person is inhaling and listen for the escape of air. Replace the seal quickly before air is sucked into the wound.

CHEST INJURIES

RIBS

IMPORTANT

- **Seek medical aid.**
- **Do not** interfere with breathing.

SYMPTOMS

The person feels pain when he inhales or when the rib area is touched.

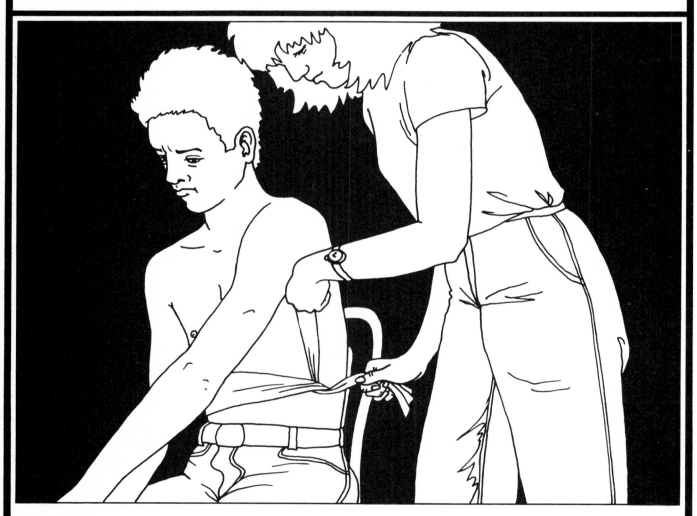

1 Restrict the movement of the chest by binding the lower half with a large bath towel or several wide cloth bandages. Place the center of the binder over the injured area and bring the ends together in a loose half-knot on the opposite side of the body.

RIBS

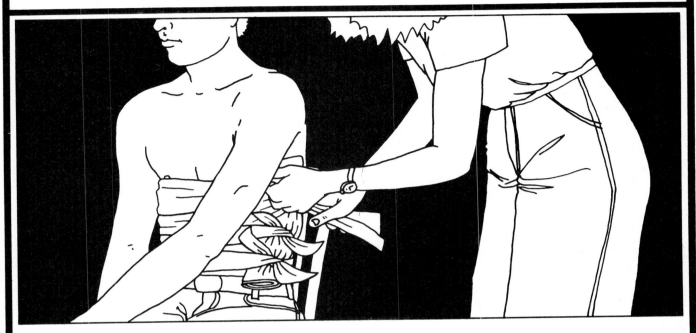

2 Use a handkerchief or other folded cloth to prevent dis-comfort from the knot, then gently tighten the half-knot. **Do not** tie too tightly. The binder should apply gentle pressure to the injured area. Take out the last slack as the person exhales.

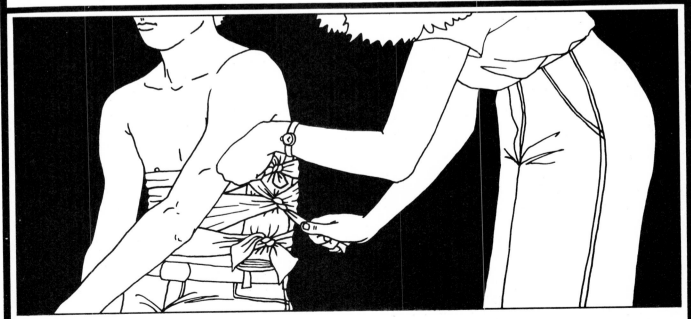

3 Complete the knot before the person starts the next breath.

CHILDBIRTH

IMPORTANT

- **Seek medical aid if childbirth seems imminent.** Until aid arrives, have the mother take short, rapid panting breaths. Tell her not to bear down, push or strain during contractions.

- **Do not** hold back the baby's head, cross the mother's legs or otherwise try to delay the birth.

- Be sure to wash your hands thoroughly before you assist the mother.

- All objects near the mother and baby should be sterile or as clean as possible.

- **Do not** touch the inside of the birth canal.

- If the umbilical cord protrudes into the birth canal before the child is born, have the mother raise her knees up toward her chest.

SYMPTOMS

Contractions every 2 minutes or more frequently. The birth opening is dilated to the size of a half-dollar. The mother feels an urge to strain or push down during contractions. She senses that the birth is imminent.

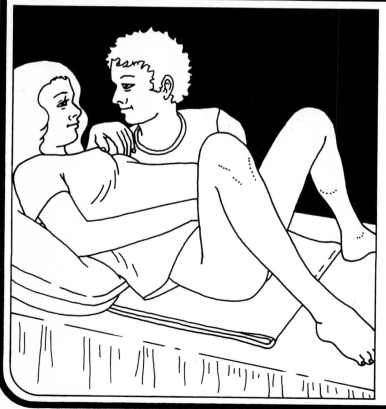

1 Take the mother to a bedroom or other warm, private area. Remove undergarments that may interfere with delivery. Have her lie down on her back on a flat surface. Place clean cloth, clothing or newspapers under her buttocks. Keep her knees bent, thighs widely apart and feet flat on the surface. Between contractions, encourage her to rest as much as possible.

CHILDBIRTH

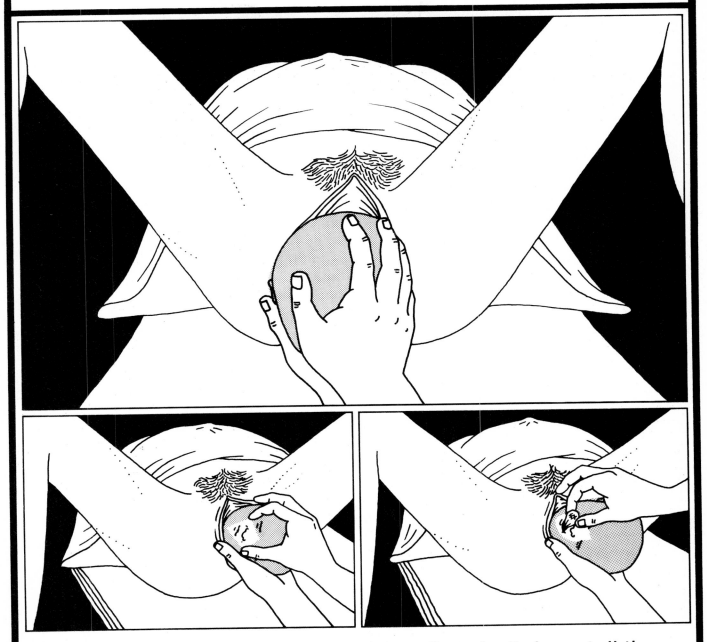

2A The baby's head should emerge first. As it does, tell the mother to stop pushing down and take shallow, panting breaths. Usually the baby's head will turn naturally over to one side. **Do not** pull or turn it. Guide and support the head, taking care to keep it away from sources of contamination. If the head is enclosed in membranes, tear them open with your fingers so the baby can breathe. As soon as possible, wipe out the baby's mouth with sterile gauze or a clean cloth.

CONTINUED ON NEXT PAGE

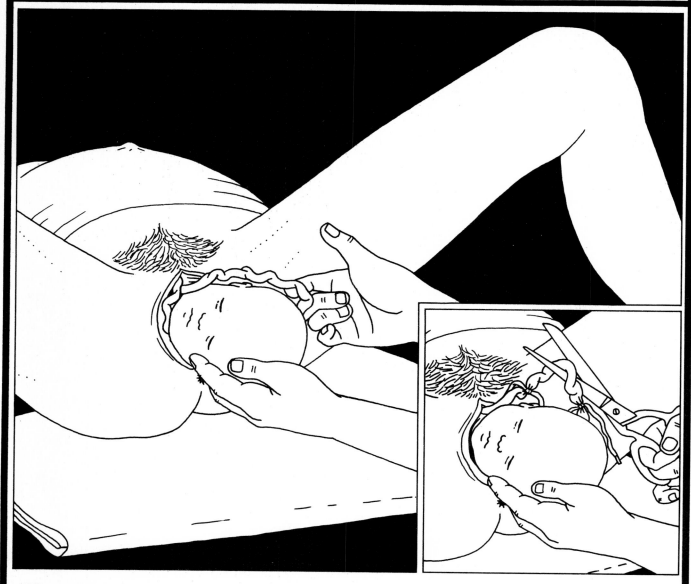

2B If the umbilical cord is wrapped around the baby's neck, place your finger between the cord and the neck and carefully unwind it by slipping it over the head. If it cannot be unwound easily, quickly tie it with white shoelaces or narrow strips of white cloth that have been boiled for 20 minutes. Make two secure double knots about 4 inches apart. Cut the cord between the two knots with a new razor blade that has been boiled in water for 20 minutes or soaked in rubbing alcohol for 10 minutes. If a razor blade isn't available, use sterilized scissors. **Do not** pull on the cord that extends from the mother's birth canal.

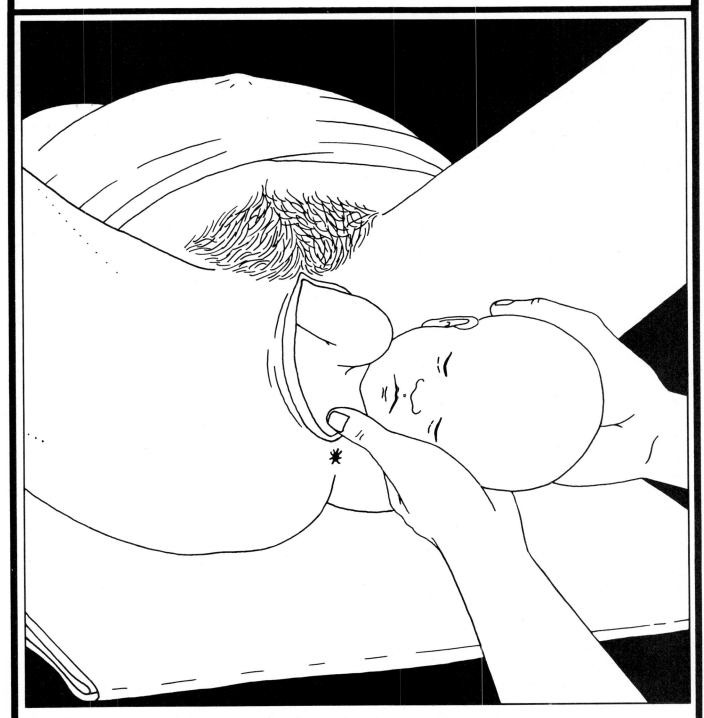

3 As the shoulders appear, lift them slightly upward while continuing to support the head and neck. The rest of the baby's body will emerge quickly. **Use extreme care to prevent the baby from slipping from your grasp. Do not** apply any tension to the umbilical cord; keep it slack.

CONTINUED ON NEXT PAGE

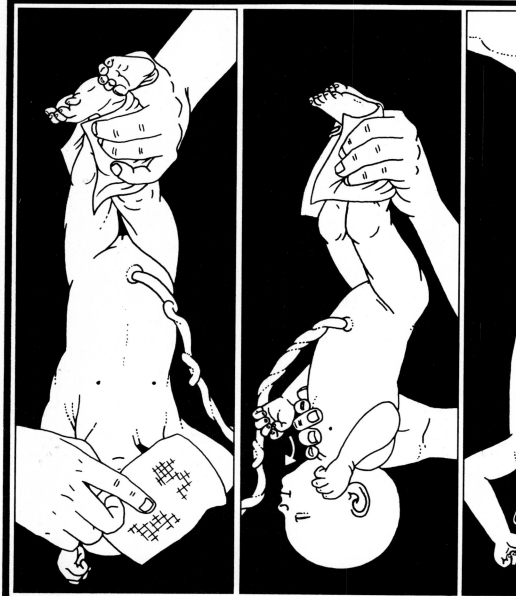
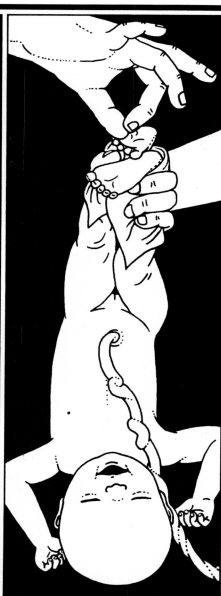

4 If the baby does not breathe immediately, lower its head and elevate its feet with your hand. Use a clean cloth to prevent slipping. Wipe out the mouth with sterile gauze, clean cloth or the like. Stroke along the neck from the chest toward the mouth with a milking motion. Wipe out the mouth again if necessary. If breathing does not begin, rub the baby's back or flick the soles of its feet with your finger. If breathing still does not begin, see **BREATHING: ARTIFICIAL RESPIRATION (INFANT & SMALL CHILD).**

5 **Do not** attempt to remove the greasy white coating on the baby's skin or to clean its eyes, nose or ears. Keep the baby warm by wrapping it in a receiving blanket. Place it on its back with a pad under its shoulders and its head extended back or put it on the mother's abdomen if she is able to hold it. If the birth canal has been torn during the birth, see **BLEEDING: CUTS & WOUNDS (DIRECT PRESSURE).**

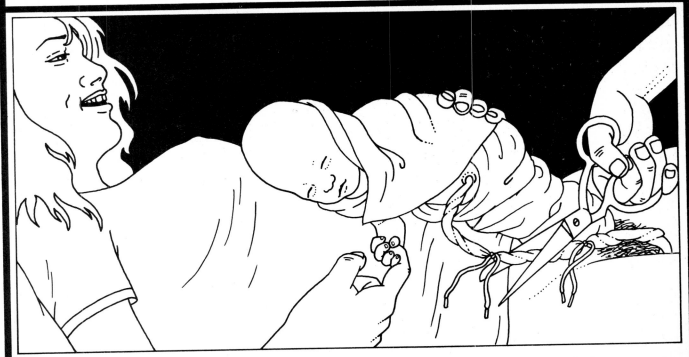

6 **Do not** cut the umbilical cord until all pulsations of the cord have stopped. This will usually be within about 5 minutes. Tie the cord with white shoelaces or narrow strips of white cloth that have been boiled for 20 minutes. Make a secure double knot about 4 inches from the baby's stomach and a second double knot about 8 inches from the baby's stomach. Cut the cord between the two sets of knots with a new razor blade that has been boiled in water for 20 minutes or soaked in rubbing alcohol for 10 minutes. If a razor blade isn't available, use sterilized scissors. **Do not** pull on the cord that extends from the mother's birth canal.

CONTINUED ON NEXT PAGE

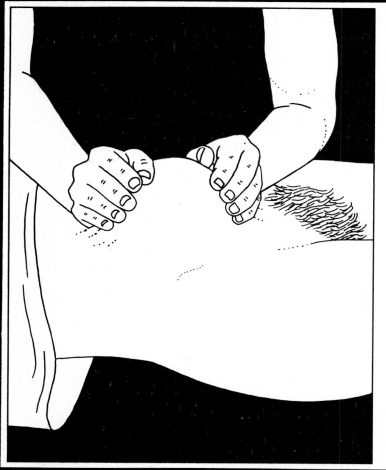

7 After a brief time, the mother will resume contractions to expel the afterbirth. **Do not** pull the cord or push the abdomen to assist her. When the afterbirth has been expelled, gently but firmly massage the mother's stomach for several minutes. Repeat the massage every 5 minutes for an hour. Save the afterbirth so it can be examined by a doctor. If contractions to expel the afterbirth do not resume within a half hour, seek medical assistance.

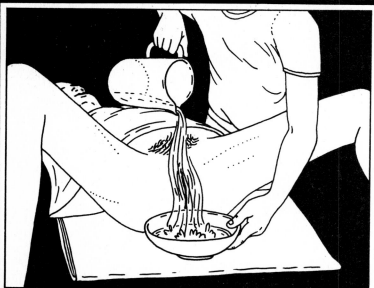

8 Cleanse the opening of the birth canal with a sterile or clean damp cloth or pour warm soapy water over it from above so that it drains towards the buttocks. Rinse with clean warm water. Cover the birth opening with a sanitary napkin, clean cloth or the like.

9 Keep the mother warm and give her fluids to drink.

CHOKING

IMPORTANT

- **Do not** interfere with the person's own efforts to free the obstruction if he can breathe, speak or cough.

- If he cannot free the obstruction, do the following:

INFANT

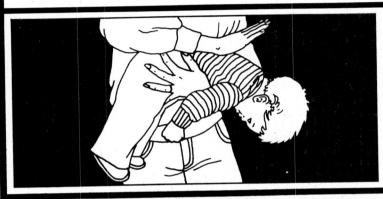

1 Place him face down on your forearm, and with the heel of the other hand, give him 4 rapid forceful blows between the shoulder blades.

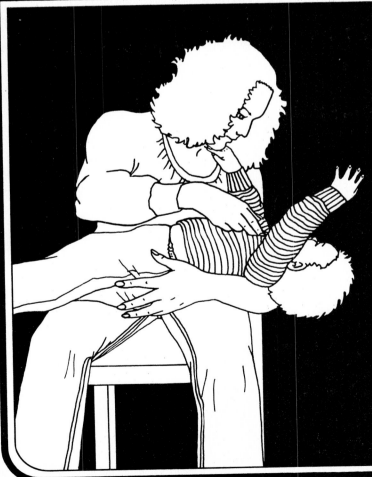

2 If the obstruction is not cleared, place him face up on your forearm with the head lower than the body. Support your arm with your thigh. Place 2 or 3 fingertips on the breastbone between the nipples and make 4 quick thrusts downward towards his chest. **Do not** thrust to either side. **Adjust the force of your thrusts to the child's size.** Repeat if necessary. Watch breathing closely. If necessary, see **BREATHING: ARTIFICIAL RESPIRATION.**

CHOKING

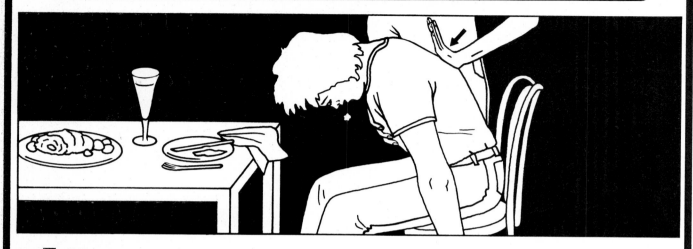

1 Have the person lower his head to chest level or lower. Support his chest with one hand, and with the heel of the other give him 4 rapid forceful blows between the shoulder blades.

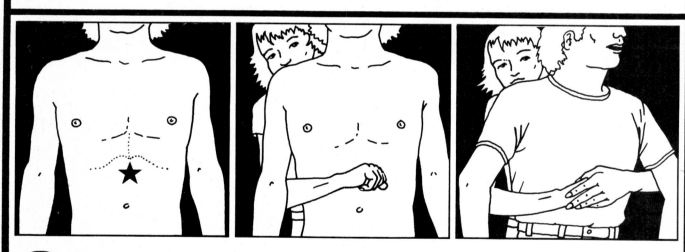

2 If the obstruction is not cleared, place your arms around the person with the thumb side of your fist against his stomach between the navel and the rib cage. Grasp your fist with your other hand and make 4 quick upward thrusts at the exact spot shown. **Do not** thrust to either side. **Adjust the force of your thrusts to the person's size.** Repeat if necessary. Watch breathing closely. If necessary, see **BREATHING: ARTIFICIAL RESPIRATION.**

CHOKING

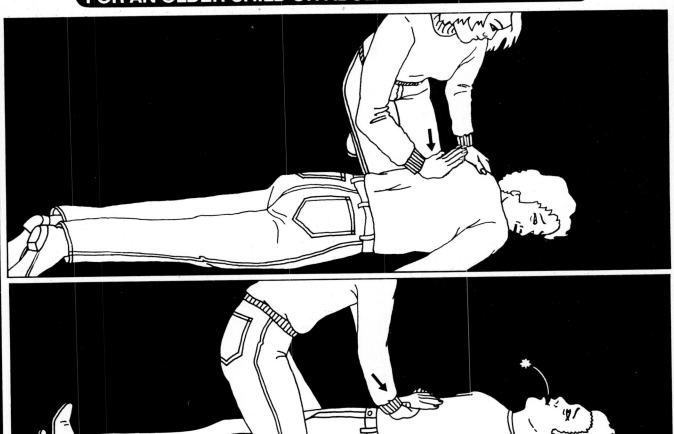

Place your knee against his chest for support, and with the heel of one hand, give him 4 rapid forceful blows between the shoulder blades. If the obstruction is not cleared, roll him on his back and kneel over his hips. Place one hand against his stomach between the navel and the rib cage. Place your other hand on top of the first. Keep your shoulders directly over his stomach and make 4 quick upward thrusts toward his chest. **Do not** thrust to either side. **Adjust the force of your thrusts to the person's size.** Repeat if necessary. Watch breathing closely. If necessary, see **BREATHING: ARTIFICIAL RESPIRATION.**

91

CHOKING

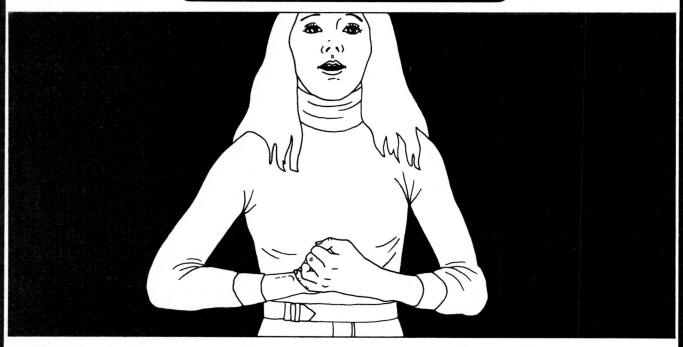

1A Press your fist against your stomach between your navel and your rib cage with a quick upward thrust.

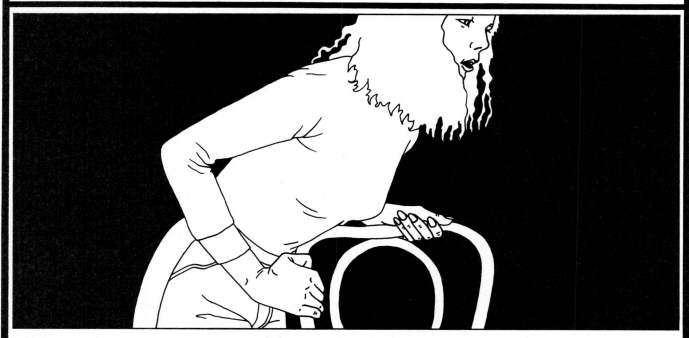

1B Or lean forward and quickly press this part of your stomach over the edge of a firm object such as a chair, sink or railing.

IMPORTANT

- **Do not** give the person anything to drink during the convulsion.

- Tell your doctor about all convulsive seizures, no matter how brief.

SYMPTOMS

Falling. Frothing at the mouth. Stiffening of the body. Jerky, uncontrollable movements. Unconsciousness.

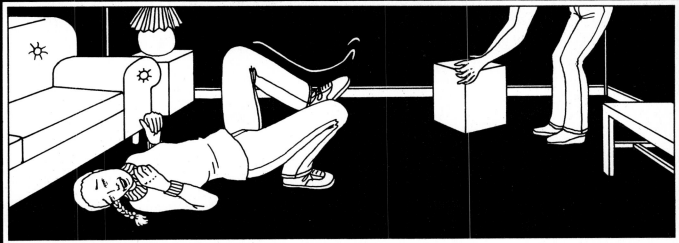

1 Clear the area of hard or sharp objects that might cause harm. Try to loosen tight clothing, but **do not** restrain the person.

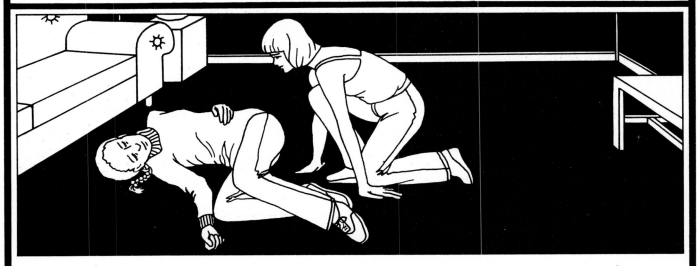

2 When the convulsion subsides, turn the person onto her side. Watch breathing closely. If necessary, see **BREATHING: ARTIFICIAL RESPIRATION.**

93

DIABETIC COMA

IMPORTANT

- **Seek medical aid immediately.**

- **Do not** give the person sugar, starch or fat in any form.

- Watch breathing closely. If necessary, see **BREATHING: ARTIFICIAL RESPIRATION.**

- **Do not** give the person anything to drink if he is unconscious.

- **Do not** mistake the sweet odor on the breath (acetone) for alcohol.

SYMPTOMS

May develop over a period of days in adults, more quickly in children. **Early symptoms may include:** Excessive thirst, appetite and urination. **May be followed by:** Weakness. Loss of appetite. Difficulty breathing. **Symptoms progress to:** Great difficulty breathing. Dry red skin and lips. Flushed appearance. Intense thirst. Characteristic sweet smell (acetone) on the breath. **May also develop:** Fever. Vomiting. Stomach pain. Confusion. Weakness. Stupor resembling drunkenness. Unconsciousness.

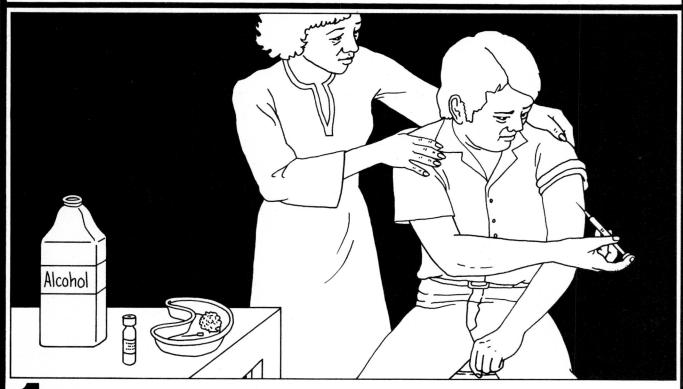

1A If insulin has been prescribed, help the person take it.

DIABETIC COMA

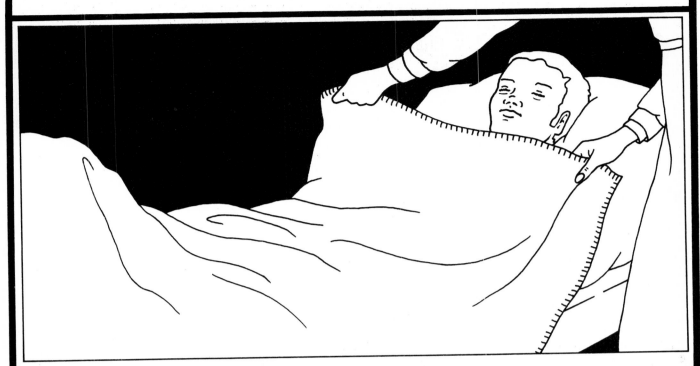

1B If not, treat for shock; see **SHOCK.**

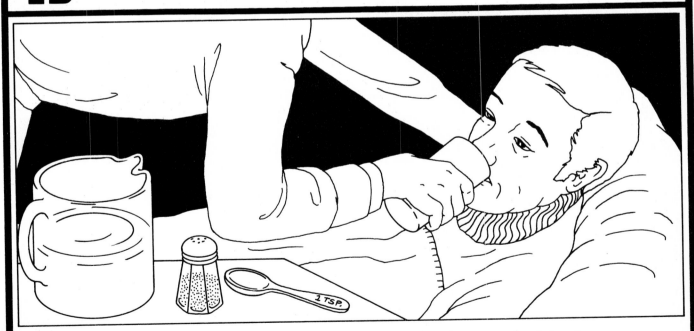

2 If the person is conscious, not vomiting and able to tolerate liquid, have him drink large quantities (up to 2 quarts) of water with salt added (1 teaspoon salt per quart). Discontinue salt water if the person becomes nauseated.

DROWNING

WATER RESCUE

- **Send for help immediately.**

- **Do not** swim to the person unless you cannot use reaching assists from land and it is a matter of life or death.

- Try to touch the person's hand or body with the reaching assist. Because of panic, he may be unaware of the assist if it doesn't touch him directly.

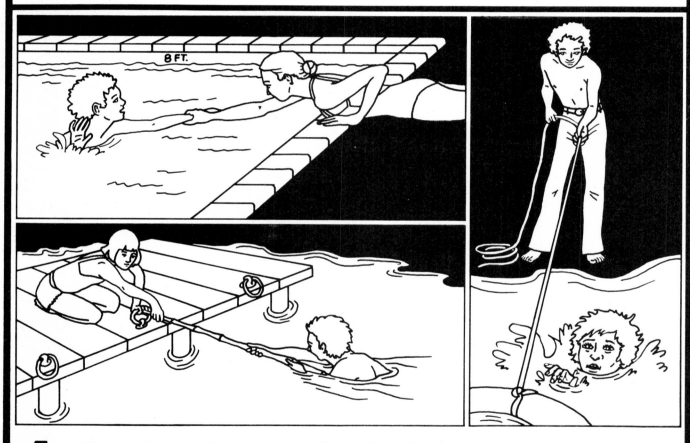

1A Try to reach the person from land with a hand, leg, clothing, pole, rope, etc. Throw him a buoy, board or anything that floats. Avoid hitting him; you may accidentally knock him unconscious. Ropes or objects attached to ropes should be thrown beyond the person, then pulled directly into his grasp. Always hold onto something with your other hand. **Do not** let the person grab you.

DROWNING

WATER RESCUE

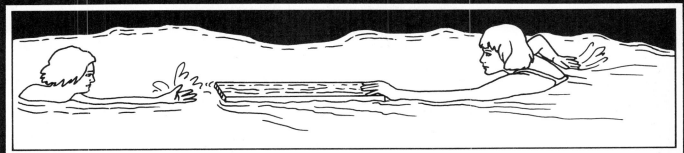

1B If he is too far to reach, wade in closer with reaching assists.

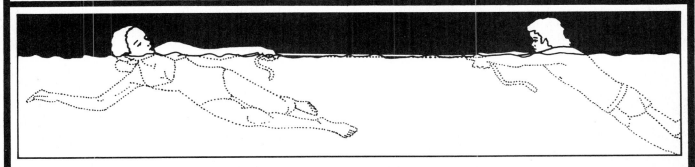

1C If you must swim to him, keep watching him or the spot you saw him last. Bring something for him to hold onto and pull him to shore. **Do not** let him grab you.

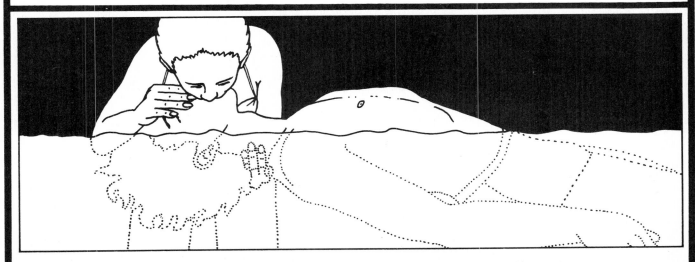

2 If necessary, begin rescue breathing immediately, even before leaving the water. See **BREATHING: ARTIFICIAL RESPIRATION.**

DROWNING

ICE RESCUE

IMPORTANT

- **Seek medical aid immediately.**

- **Do not** walk near the open ice.

- Tell the person not to try to climb out but to slide his arms onto the ice and hold on until you reach him.

- When safely back on firm footing, watch the person's breathing closely. If necessary, begin rescue breathing immediately. See **BREATHING: ARTIFICIAL RESPIRATION.**

- Treat for shock; see **SHOCK.**

- Observe for hypothermia, even if the person was in the water for only a short time; see **HYPOTHERMIA.**

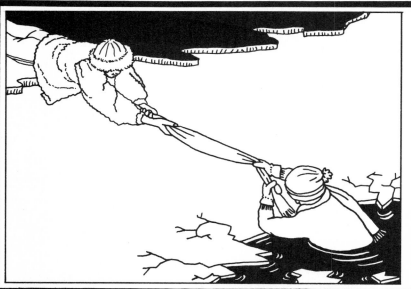

1A Try to reach the person from land with a hand, leg, clothing, rope, ladder, sled, board, etc. Tell him to hold onto the reaching assist and slide on his stomach — **not** walk upright — back to firm footing.

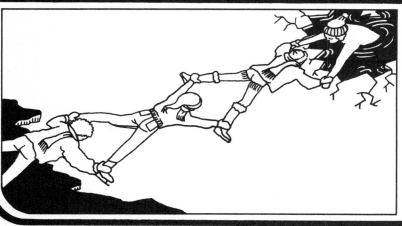

1B If necessary, form a human chain. Each person lies spread-eagled on the ice, holding the ankles of the person in front of him.

ICE RESCUE

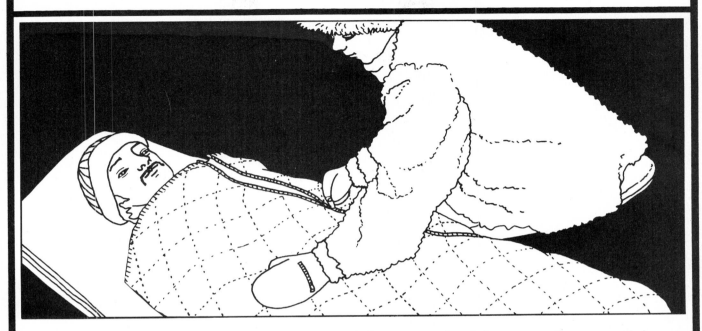

2 Quickly but gently remove his wet clothing and warm him with blankets, a sleeping bag, etc. Observe for hypothermia; see **HYPOTHERMIA.**

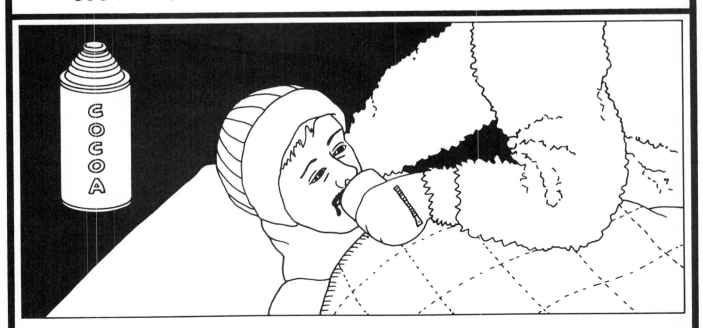

3 If immersion was less than 10 minutes and there are no symptoms of hypothermia, give him a warm sweetened drink. Check for frostbite; see **FROSTBITE.**

EAR INJURIES

FOREIGN OBJECTS & CUTS

IMPORTANT

- If the ear is severed, see **BLEEDING: CUTS & WOUNDS (AMPUTATIONS).**

- Blood or clear fluid coming from the ear suggests a serious injury to the head; see **HEAD INJURIES.**

FOREIGN OBJECTS

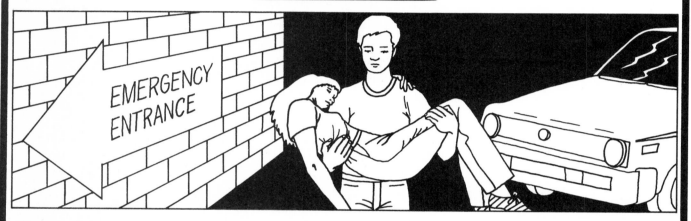

Turn the person's head onto the injured side, then **seek medical aid immediately. Do not** try to remove the object yourself.

CUTS

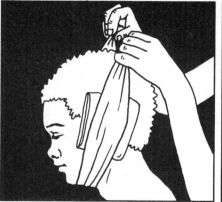 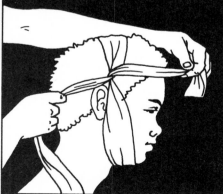 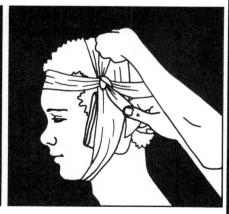

Control the bleeding by pressing gauze or a clean cloth directly over the wound and elevating the person's head. Apply a wide bandage to maintain the pressure.

EAR INJURIES

PERFORATED EARDRUM

IMPORTANT

- **Seek medical aid immediately.**

- If the person has received a blow to the head, check for symptoms of serious head injuries before treating the ear; see **HEAD INJURIES (CLOSED HEAD INJURIES).**

- **Do not** insert drops, fingers or instruments into the ear if you suspect a perforated eardrum.

- **Do not** permit the person to hit the side of his head in an effort to restore lost hearing.

SYMPTOMS

Sudden severe pain. Reduction in hearing. Ringing in the ears. Possible dizziness. Possible blood or fluid draining from the ear.

IF PERFORATION HAS BEEN CAUSED BY A BLOW TO THE HEAD

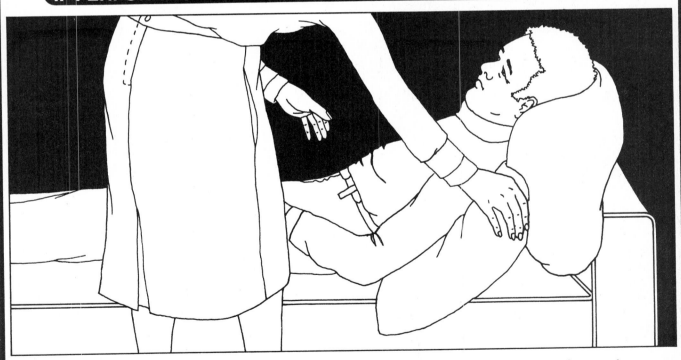

1 Keep the person lying down. If there is no sign of neck injury, place a pillow, jacket, etc. under both his head and shoulders, **not** his head alone.

CONTINUED ON NEXT PAGE

PERFORATED EARDRUM
CONTINUED

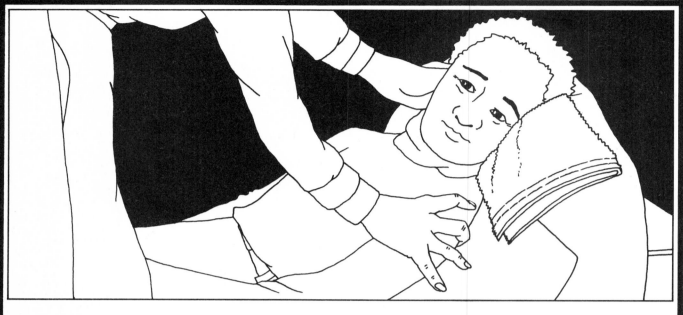

2 Turn the head toward the affected side so fluids may drain from the ear. **Do not** stop the flow of fluid or clean the ear canal.

IF PERFORATION HAS NOT BEEN CAUSED BY A BLOW TO THE HEAD

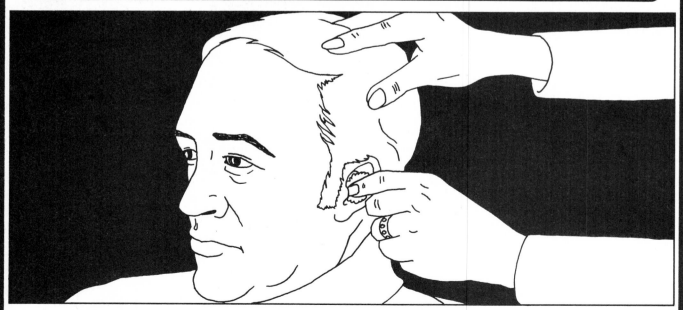

Place a piece of gauze loosely in the outer ear canal.

ELECTRIC SHOCK

IMPORTANT

- **Do not** touch the person directly while he remains in contact with the current.

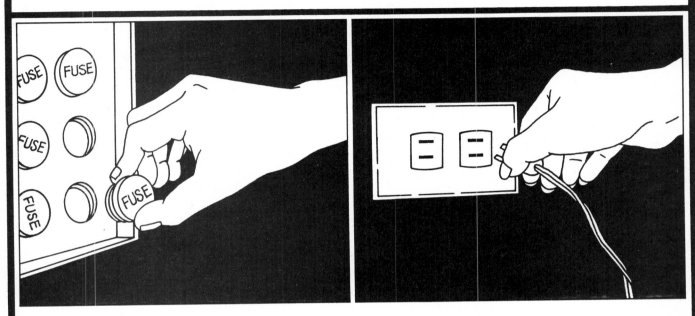

1A Try to turn off the current by removing the fuse or unplugging the electrical cord from the outlet.

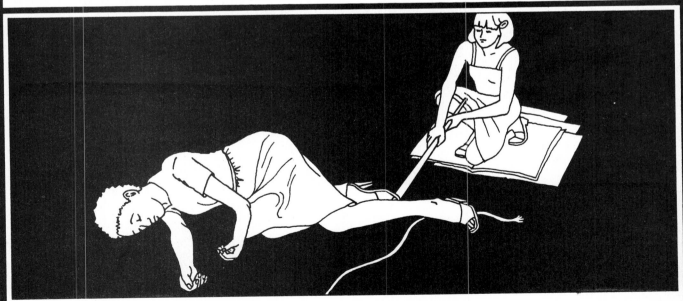

1B If that isn't possible, stand on something dry — a blanket, rubber mat, newspapers, etc. — and push the person or the wire away with a dry board or pole.

CONTINUED ON NEXT PAGE

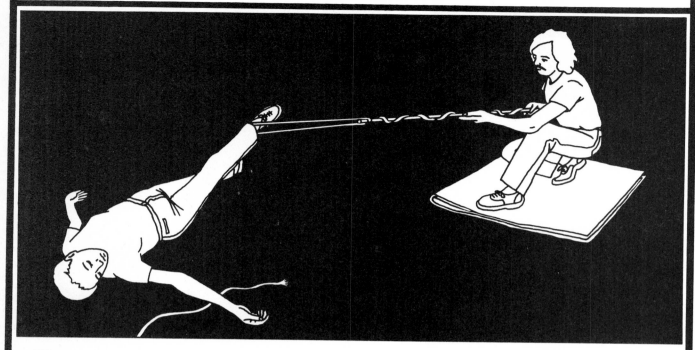

1c Or pull the person away with a dry rope looped over the foot or arm.

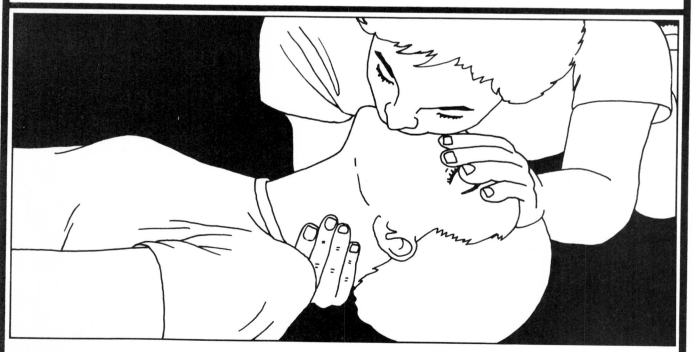

2 If necessary, begin rescue breathing immediately; see **BREATHING: ARTIFICIAL RESPIRATION.** Treat for shock; see **SHOCK.** Also treat for burns; see **BURNS.**

EYE INJURIES

CHEMICALS IN THE EYE

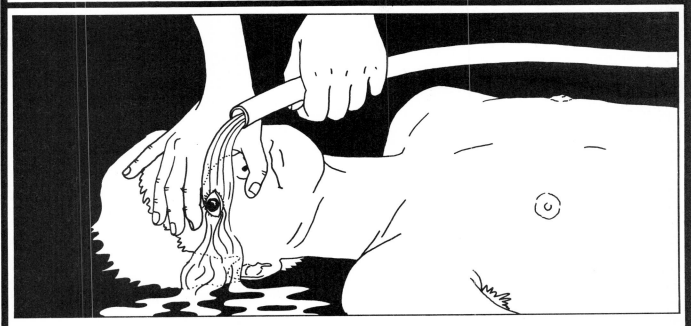

1 Holding the eyelid open, flush the eye immediately with gently running water for at least 5 minutes. **Do not** let the water run into the other eye.

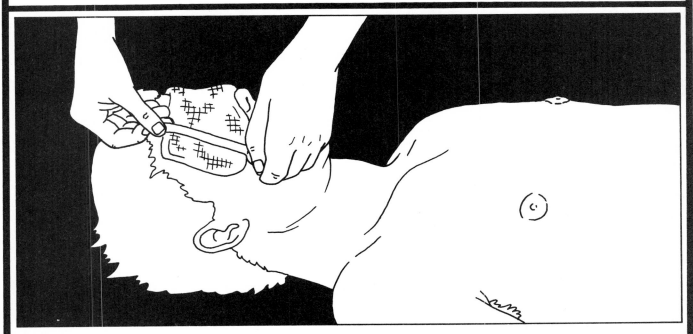

2 Apply gauze or a clean cloth. Hold it in place with a loosely fastened bandage that covers both eyes. **Seek medical aid.**

EYE INJURIES

EYELID, EYEBALL & IMPALED OBJECTS

IMPORTANT

- **Seek medical aid immediately.**
- **Do not** wash out the eye.
- If you must move the person, use a stretcher. See **TRANSPORTING THE INJURED.**

LACERATED EYELID

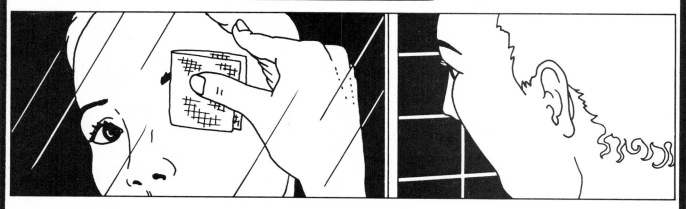

Control the bleeding with a pressure dressing or direct pressure against the lid and bone.

LACERATED EYEBALL

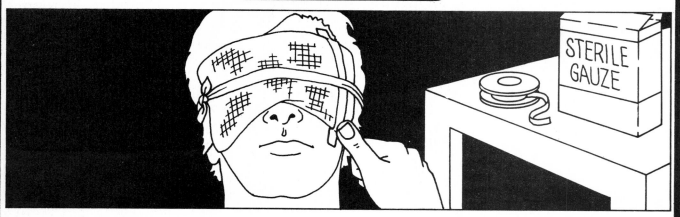

Cover **both** eyes loosely with gauze or a clean cloth. **Do not** apply pressure. If necessary, secure the person's hands so he cannot touch his eyes.

EYE INJURIES

EYELID, EYEBALL & IMPALED OBJECTS

IMPALED OBJECTS

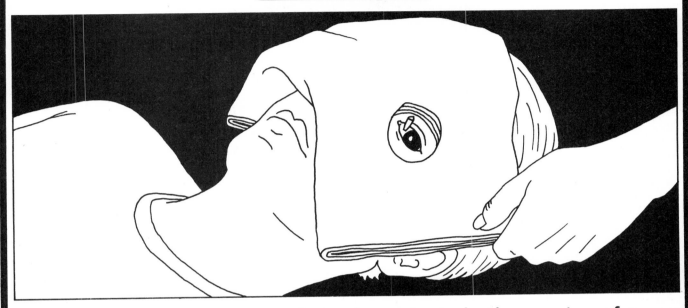

1 **Do not** try to remove. Cut a large hole in the center of a thick dressing, and apply the dressing carefully so it doesn't touch the eye or object.

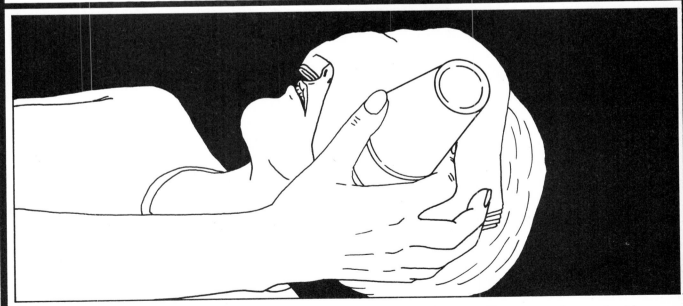

2 Place a paper cup or cone over the eye. **Do not** touch the eye itself.

CONTINUED ON NEXT PAGE

EYE INJURIES

EYELID, EYEBALL & IMPALED OBJECTS
CONTINUED

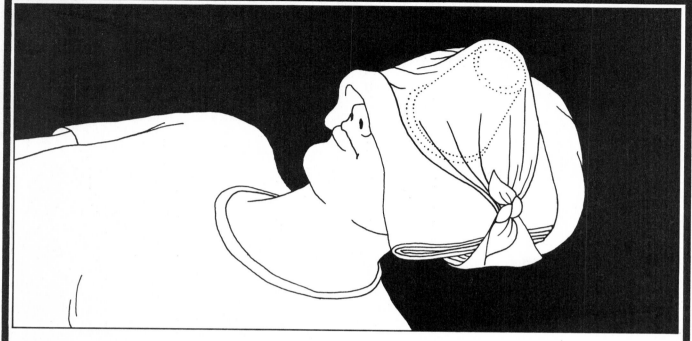

3 Secure the cup in place with a gauze or clean cloth dressing. Bandage both eyes to prevent movement in the injured eye.

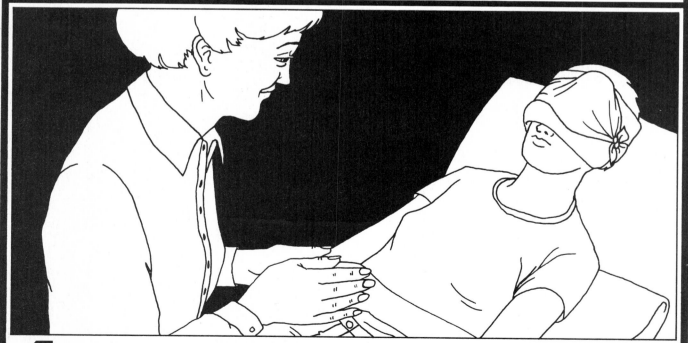

4 Keep the person calm and offer reassurance.

EYE INJURIES

FOREIGN OBJECTS

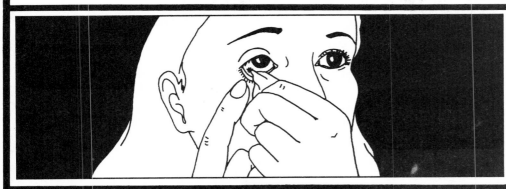

LOWER EYELID

Remove with a clean handkerchief or cloth.

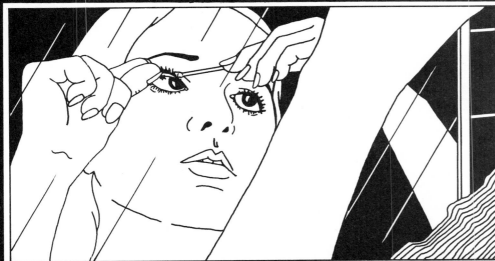

UPPER EYELID

1 Clasp the upper lash between your thumb and forefinger, then fold it back over an applicator swab.

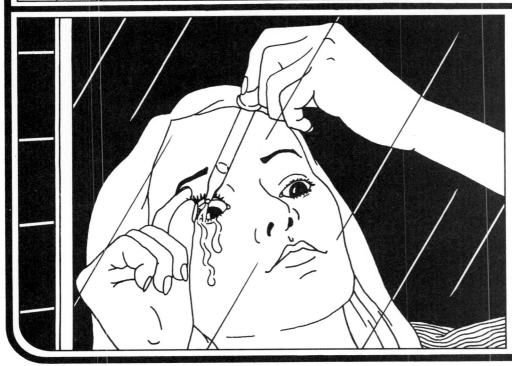

2 Have the person look down to expose the upper surface of the eyeball, then wash out the eye with water, letting the water drain down and away from the eye.

FAINTING

IMPORTANT

- If possible, prevent the person from falling to the floor. At the first indication of weakness or faintness, help him sit down.

- **Seek medical aid.** Tell your doctor about all periods of unconsciousness, no matter how brief.

- Watch breathing closely. If necessary, see **BREATHING: ARTIFICIAL RESPIRATION.**

- **If the person is unconscious, do not** give him anything to drink.

- If the person has fallen, check for injuries which may have resulted.

SYMPTOMS

Brief, sudden partial or total loss of consciousness, followed by complete recovery. May occur as a result of remaining in one position for an extended period or from pain, illness, anxiety or other emotional stress. **Early symptoms may include:** Paleness. Sweating. Nausea. Dizziness.

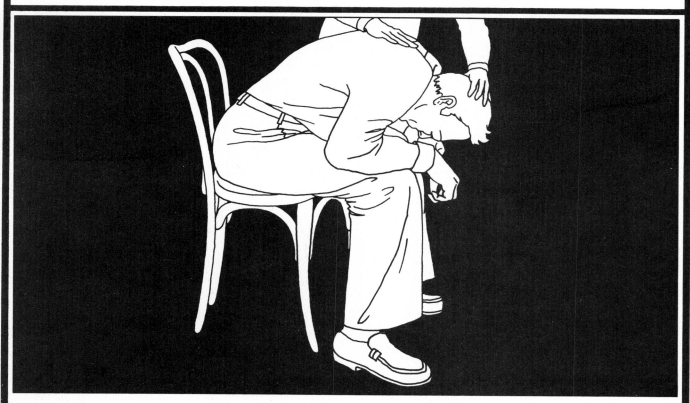

1A If the person is conscious and seated, place his head between his knees.

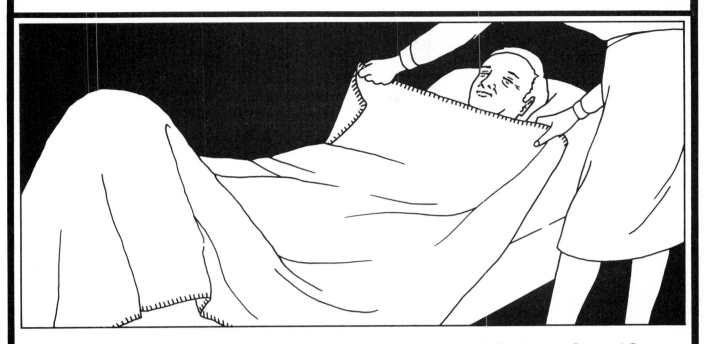

1B Otherwise, lay him down and elevate his legs 8 to 12 inches. If he vomits, turn his head to the side or roll him onto his side to keep the airway open.

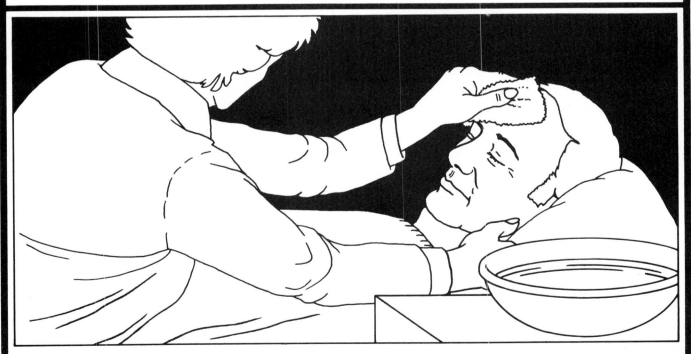

2 Loosen tight clothing and provide good ventilation. Bathe the person's face with cool water. **Do not** permit him to stand or walk until recovery is complete.

FEVER

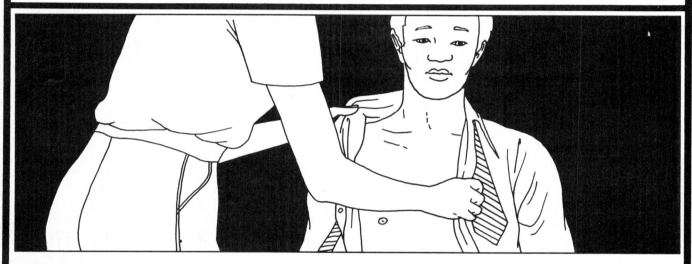

1 Undress the person in a cool (**not cold**) well-ventilated room. Avoid drafts and chilling.

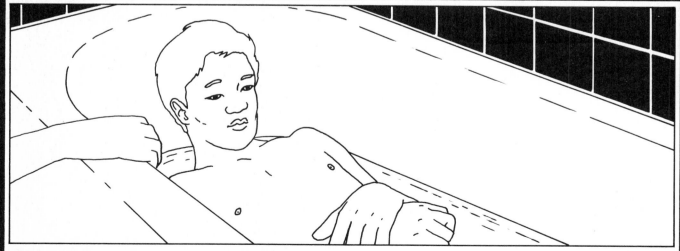

2 Place him in a partially filled tub of lukewarm water, keeping most of his body exposed to the air.

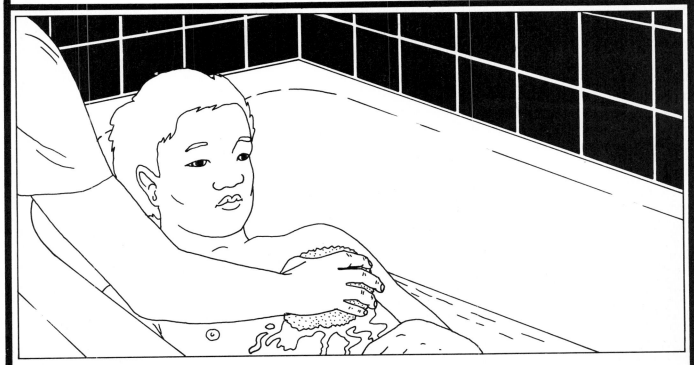

3 Sponge his entire body with light, brisk strokes for 15 to 20 minutes. (If a tub isn't handy, use a sponge bath.)

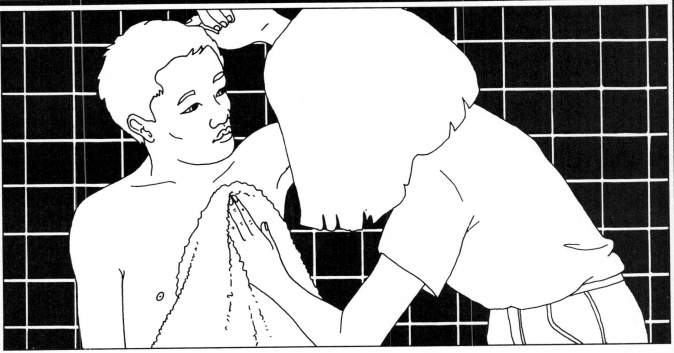

4 Dry the person vigorously. Watch his temperature closely, and repeat cooling if necessary.

FROSTBITE

IMPORTANT

- **Seek medical aid immediately.**
- **Do not** rub or massage affected areas.
- **Do not** apply hot water or strong heat.
- **Do not** break blisters.
- **Do not** give the person anything alcoholic to drink.

SYMPTOMS

Usually affects the fingers, toes, ears, nose or cheeks. The skin looks glossy and white or grayish yellow and is hard to the touch. Blisters may develop. Pain, changing to feeling of intense cold or numbness.

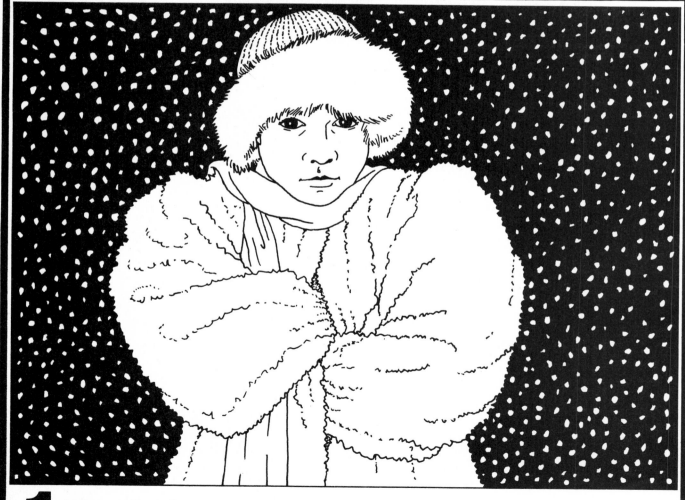

1 Warm the frozen parts against the body.

FROSTBITE

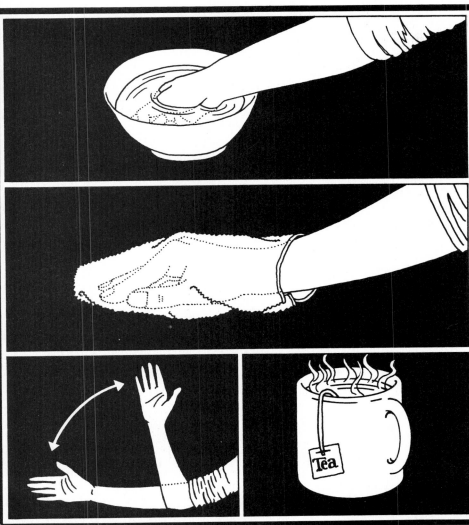

2 Take the person indoors. Remove clothing restricting circulation. Immerse frozen parts in warm (**not hot**) water, or cover lightly with warm towels or blankets. Discontinue warming when parts become flushed. Raise and lower affected limbs to stimulate circulation. Give the person warm soup, tea, etc.

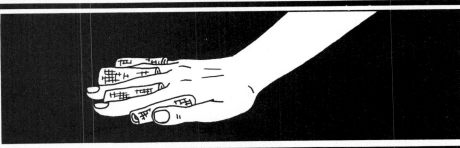

3 Keep affected toes or fingers separated with dry gauze or clean cloth.

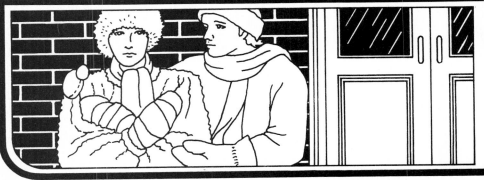

4 If the person must go to the hospital, loosely bandage the affected areas.

HEAD INJURIES

CLOSED HEAD INJURIES

IMPORTANT

- Closed head injuries may be more severe than they seem. To be safe, **call your doctor immediately.**

- Watch breathing closely. If necessary, see **BREATHING: ARTIFICIAL RESPIRATION.**

- **Do not** move the person unless absolutely necessary. If you must move him, see **TRANSPORTING THE INJURED.**

- If the person is unconscious, assume there is a neck injury. See **BACK & NECK INJURIES.** Note how long he remains unconscious.

- Treat for shock; see **SHOCK.**

SYMPTOMS

Unconsciousness. Difficulty breathing. Vomiting. Convulsions. Clear fluid or blood running from ears, nose or mouth. Paralysis of any part of the body. Loss of bowel or bladder control. Unequal pupils. Skull deformity.

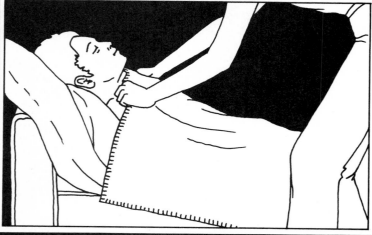

1 Keep the person lying down. If there is no sign of neck injury, place a pillow, jacket, etc. under **both** his head and his shoulders, **not** his head alone. If there are signs of neck injury, see **BACK & NECK INJURIES.**

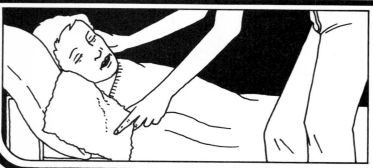

2 Turn his head to one side so fluids may drain from his mouth. **Seek medical aid immediately.**

HEAD INJURIES

OPEN HEAD INJURIES

IMPORTANT

- **Seek medical aid immediately.** Head injuries may be more severe than they seem.

- **Do not** attempt to clean deep scalp wounds of foreign matter.

- For serious head wounds, treat for shock; see **SHOCK.**

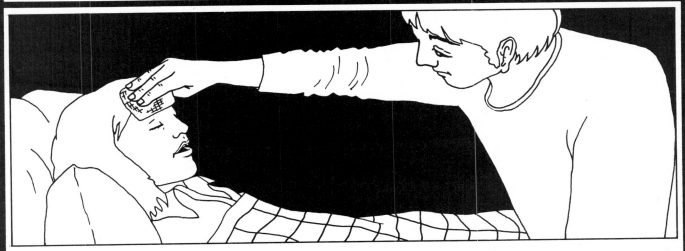

1 Control bleeding by raising the person's head and shoulders higher than her heart. **Do not** bend her neck.

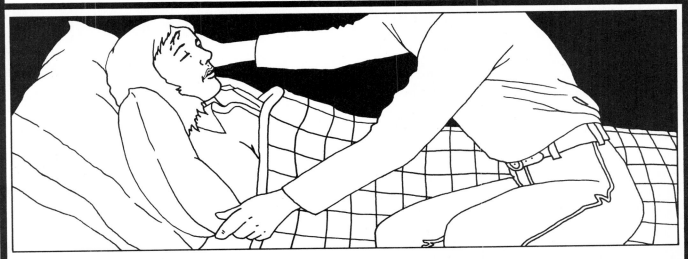

2 Further control bleeding by lightly pressing gauze or a clean cloth on the wound. Use several layers of dressing, if necessary. Avoid heavy pressure.

CONTINUED ON NEXT PAGE

OPEN HEAD INJURIES
CONTINUED

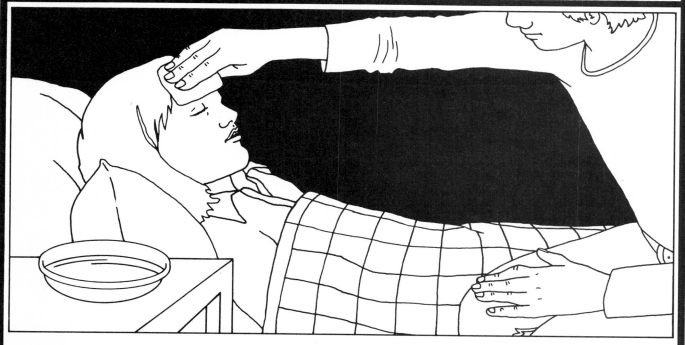

3 Clean minor head wounds carefully. Wipe **away** from the wound, **not** toward it.

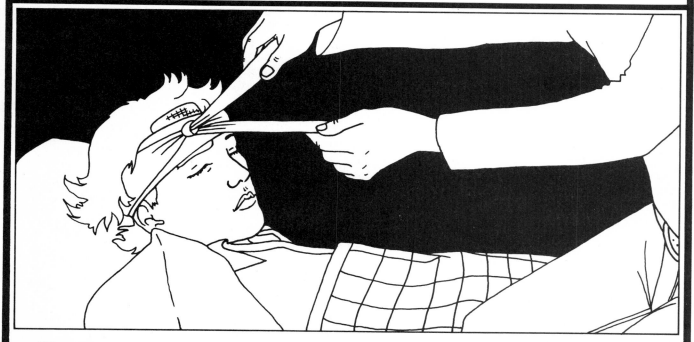

4 When bleeding is under control, bandage the dressing in place.

HEAD INJURIES

IMPALED OBJECTS: CHEEK & SKULL

IMPORTANT

- Seek medical aid immediately.

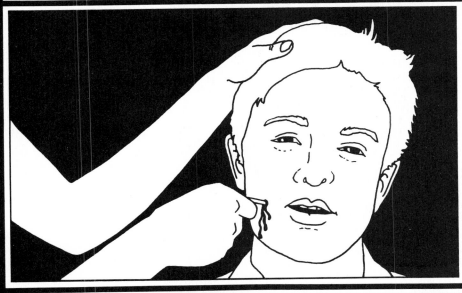

CHEEK

1 Try to remove the object by pulling it carefully from the angle it entered the cheek. **Do not force. (For an impaled fishhook, seek medical aid.)**

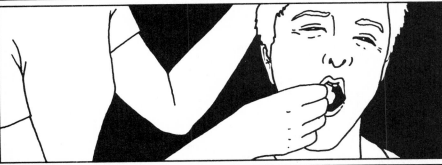

2 Control the bleeding by packing the inside of the cheek with gauze or a clean cloth.

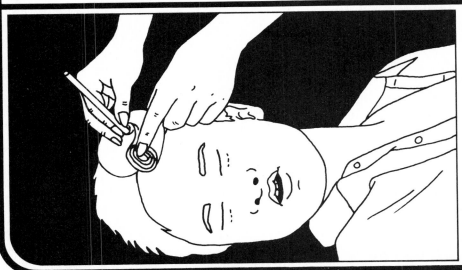

SKULL

Do not remove an impaled object from the skull. See **BLEEDING: CUTS & WOUNDS (IMPALED OBJECTS).**

HEAD INJURIES

FACE & JAW

IMPORTANT

- **Seek medical aid.**
- Remove all broken teeth and foreign matter from the person's mouth. Save the teeth for possible replanting.
- Treat for shock; see **SHOCK.**

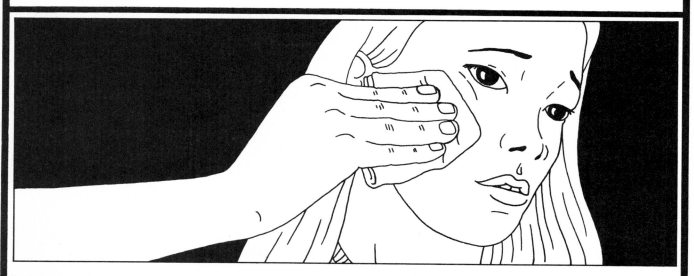

1A Raise the head higher than the heart, then control bleeding through direct pressure with gauze or a clean cloth.

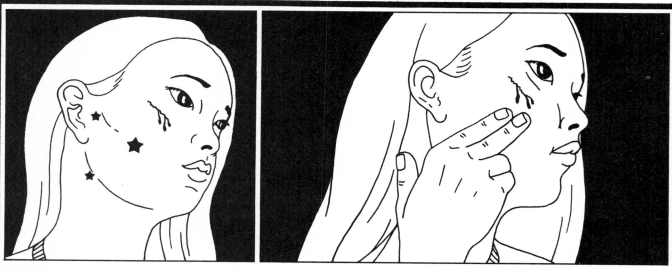

1B If necessary, also press the indicated pressure point until bleeding is brought under control.

FACE & JAW

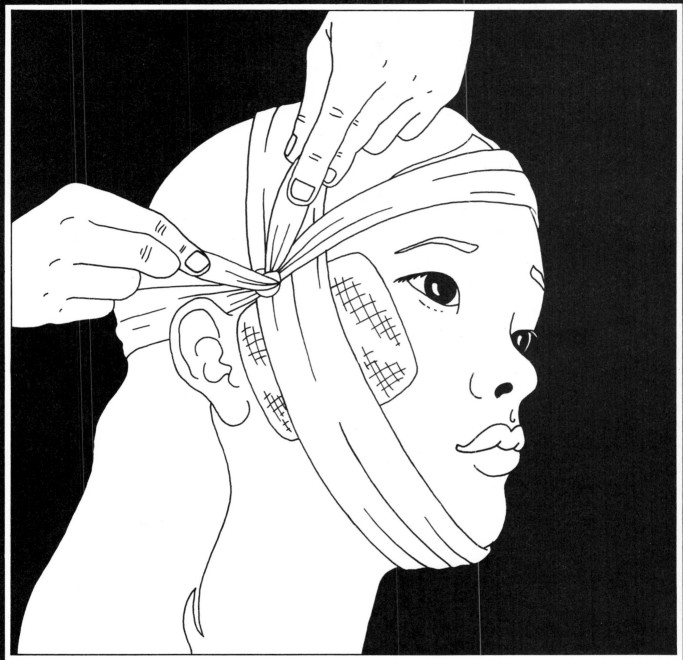

2 Apply a clean dressing or cloth, and hold it in place with a bandage.

For a jaw injury, **seek medical aid immediately. Do not** move the jaw.

HEART ATTACK

IMPORTANT

- **Send for an ambulance and oxygen immediately** if symptoms last more than 2 minutes, even if the person claims to be fine.

- Observe for shock; see **SHOCK.**

SYMPTOMS

Persistent or intermittent pain or pressure at the center of the chest, which may radiate to the shoulders, arms, neck or jaw. May include: Extreme shortness of breath. Anxiety. Sweating. Pale or bluish lips, gums, skin and fingernails.

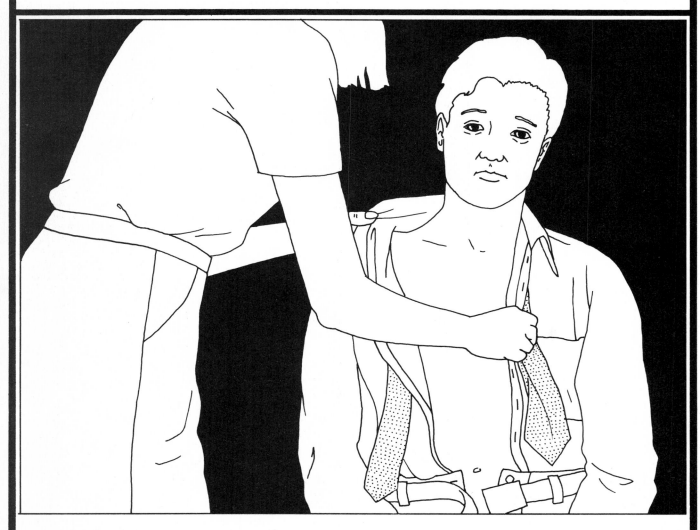

1A Place the person in the most comfortable position and loosen his clothing. Provide good ventilation but avoid chilling.

HEART ATTACK

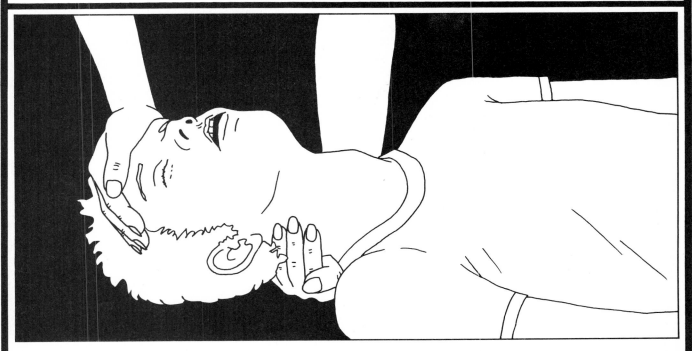

1B If he is unconscious, place him on his back and tilt his head back to open his air passage. Check his breathing closely.

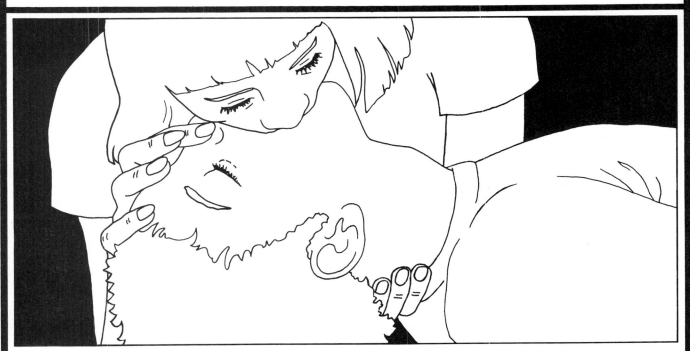

2 If necessary, start rescue breathing immediately. See **BREATHING: ARTIFICIAL RESPIRATION.** If breathing does not resume and there is no pulse, see **HEART FAILURE.**

HEART FAILURE

INFANT

IMPORTANT

- **Send for an ambulance and oxygen immediately.**

- Because first aid for heart failure is difficult and potentially dangerous, it is best administered by someone who has been fully trained in the procedure. However, if a trained person is not present or you are alone, you must begin first aid immediately since the alternative is death.

- **Waste no time, but be certain all symptoms are present before starting first aid.** To check unconsciousness, call the infant loudly, tap him on the shoulder or shake him gently. Check the pulse slowly and carefully on the inside of the upper arm. It is extremely important to find the pulse if one is present. Take between 5 and 10 seconds to find it. **Do not** rush. It is easily missed under emergency conditions.

SYMPTOMS

Unconsciousness. No breathing. No pulse.

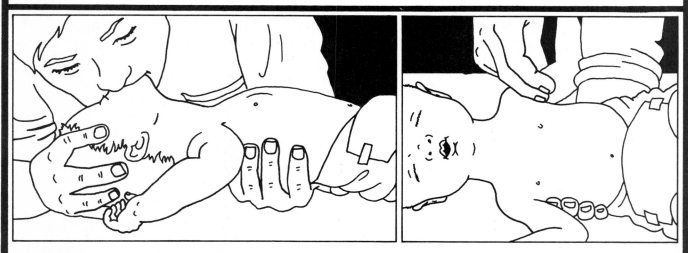

1 Place the infant on his back on a firm surface and gently tip back his head. Look and listen for air leaving his lungs. If breathing does not resume, put your open mouth over his nose and mouth, forming an airtight seal, and give 4 quick, gentle puffs of air. Recheck all symptoms. If pulse has started, see **BREATHING: ARTIFICIAL RESPIRATION.** If pulse has not started, then:

HEART FAILURE

INFANT

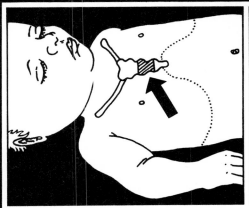 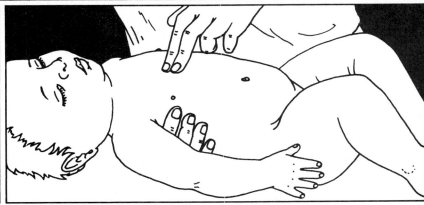

2 Place the tips of your index and middle finger on the exact spot shown. (**Do not** press the lower end of the sternum.) Support the infant's back by placing your other hand under his shoulders.

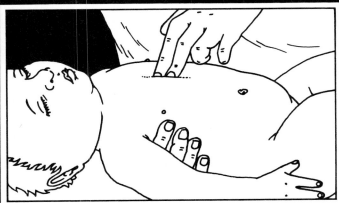 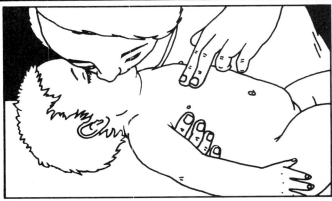

3 Make short, smooth thrusts directly downward about ½ to 1 inch, 100 times a minute. After every 5 compressions, breathe into the infant's mouth (using short gentle puffs of air) as your fingertips begin to rise. Give the infant one new breath every 3 seconds, 20 a minute. (**Do not** remove fingertips between compressions.) If breathing seems blocked, see **CHOKING,** then resume first aid. Discontinue compressions when the heartbeat is restored; continue rescue breathing until the infant breathes spontaneously or professional help arrives.

CHILD

IMPORTANT

- **Send for an ambulance and oxygen immediately.**

- Because first aid for heart failure is difficult and potentially dangerous, it is best administered by someone who has been fully trained in the procedure. However, if a trained person is not present or you are alone, you must begin first aid immediately since the alternative is death.

- **Waste no time, but be certain all symptoms are present before starting first aid.** To check unconsciousness, call the child loudly, tap her on the shoulder or shake her gently. Check the pulse slowly and carefully at the large artery of the neck. It is extremely important to find the pulse if one is present. Take between 5 and 10 seconds to find it. **Do not** rush. It is easily missed under emergency conditions.

- If possible, have one person perform rescue breathing and another administer heart compressions. If alone, you will have to do both simultaneously.

SYMPTOMS

Unconsciousness. No breathing. No pulse.

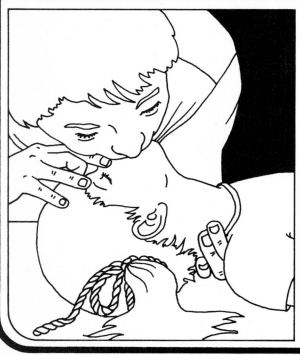

1 Place the child on her back on a firm surface and gently tip back her head. Look and listen for air leaving her lungs. If breathing does not resume, open her mouth and pinch her nose closed. Put your open mouth over her mouth, forming an airtight seal, and give 4 quick, gentle breaths. Recheck all symptoms. If pulse has started, see **BREATHING: ARTIFICIAL RESPIRATION.** If pulse has not started, then:

HEART FAILURE

CHILD

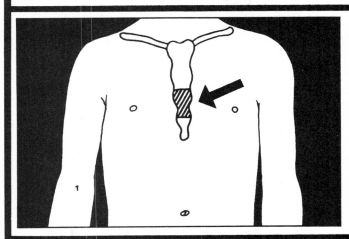

2 Place the heel of one hand about 2 finger-widths above the tip of the sternum. (**Do not** press the tip.) Your fingertips should be pointing directly across the child's body but not pressing against the ribs.

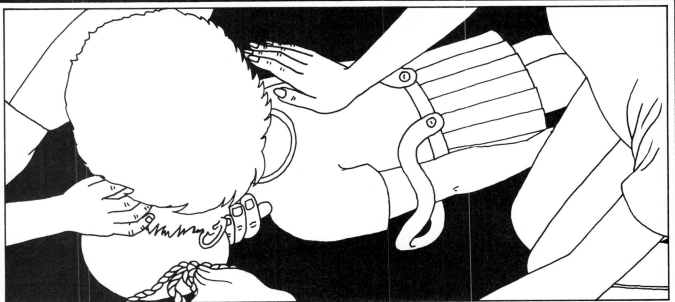

3A **If you have assistance:** make short, smooth thrusts directly downward about 1 to 1½ inches, 80 times a minute. After every 5 compressions, have your assistant breathe gently into the child's mouth as the heel of your hand begins to rise, giving the child one new breath every 4 seconds, 15 a minute. (**Do not** remove your hand between compressions.) If breathing seems blocked, see **CHOKING,** then resume first aid. Discontinue compressions when the heartbeat is restored; continue rescue breathing until the child breathes spontaneously or professional help arrives.

CONTINUED ON NEXT PAGE

CHILD
CONTINUED

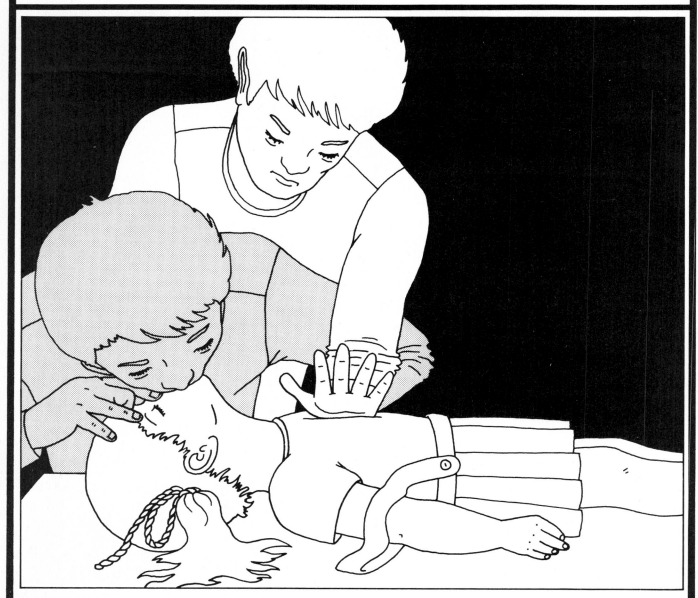

3B **If you are alone:** Make short, smooth thrusts directly downward about 1 to 1½ inches, 80 times a minute. After every 5 compressions give the child a quick breath. (**Do not** remove your hand between compressions.) If breathing seems blocked, see **CHOKING,** then resume first aid. Discontinue compressions when the heartbeat is restored; continue rescue breathing until the child breathes spontaneously or professional help arrives.

HEART FAILURE

OLDER CHILD & ADULT

(IMPORTANT)

- **Send for an ambulance and oxygen immediately.**

- Because first aid for heart failure is difficult and potentially dangerous, it is best administered by someone who has been fully trained in the procedure. However, if a trained person is not present or you are alone, you must begin first aid immediately since the alternative is death.

- **Waste no time, but be certain all symptoms are present before starting first aid.** To check unconsciousness, call the person loudly, tap her on the shoulder or shake her gently. Check the pulse slowly and carefully at the large artery of the neck. It is extremely important to find the pulse if one is present. Take between 5 to 10 seconds to find it. **Do not** rush. It is easily missed under emergency conditions.

- If possible, have one person perform rescue breathing and another administer heart compressions. If alone, you will have to do both simultaneously.

(SYMPTOMS)

Unconsciousness. No breathing. No pulse.

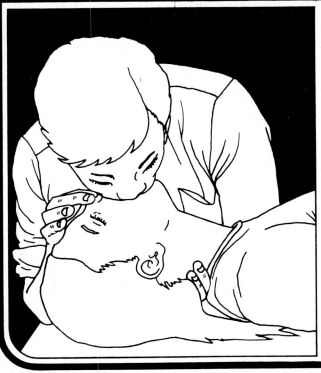

1 Place the person on her back on a firm surface and gently tip back her head. Look and listen for air leaving her lungs. If breathing does not resume, open her mouth and pinch her nose closed. Put your open mouth over her mouth, forming an airtight seal, and give 4 quick, full breaths. Recheck all symptoms. If pulse has started, see **BREATHING: ARTIFICIAL RESPIRATION.** If pulse has not started, then:

CONTINUED ON NEXT PAGE

OLDER CHILD & ADULT
CONTINUED

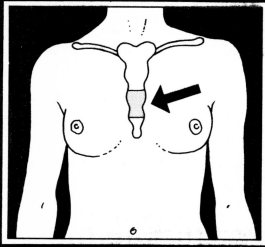

2 Place the heel of one hand about 2 finger-widths above the tip of the sternum. (**Do not** press the tip.) Your fingertips should be pointing directly across the person's body but not pressing against the ribs. Place your other hand on top of the first. Keep your elbows straight and your shoulders directly over your hands.

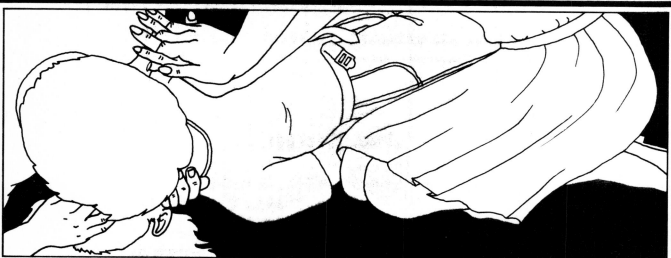

3A **If you have assistance:** Make short, smooth thrusts directly downward about 1½ to 2 inches, 60 times a minute. After every 5 compressions, have your assistant take a deep breath and breathe fully into the person's mouth as the heels of your hands begin to rise, giving the person one new breath every 5 seconds, 12 a minute. (**Do not** remove your hands between compressions.) If breathing seems blocked, see **CHOKING,** then resume first aid. Discontinue compressions when the heartbeat is restored; continue rescue breathing until the person breathes spontaneously or professional help arrives.

HEART FAILURE

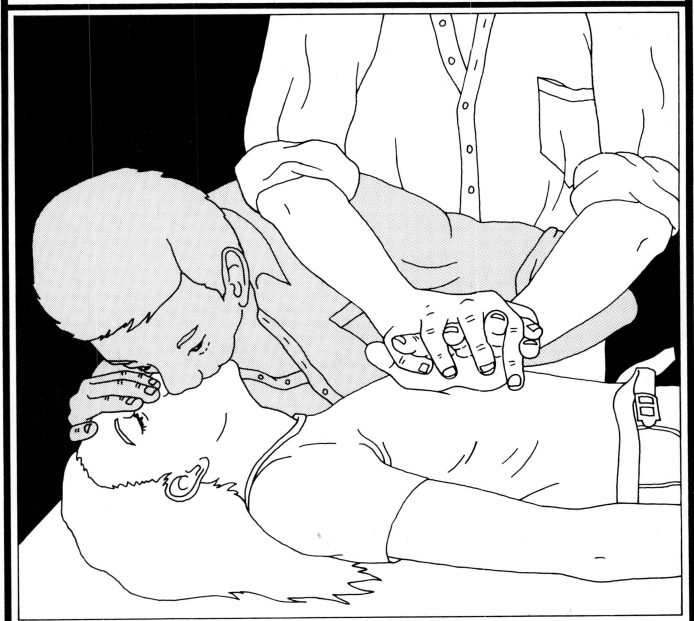

3B **If you are alone:** Make short, smooth thrusts directly downward about 1½ to 2 inches, 80 times a minute. After every 15 compressions, give 2 quick breaths. If breathing seems blocked, see **CHOKING,** then resume first aid. Discontinue compressions when the heartbeat is restored; continue rescue breathing until the person breathes spontaneously or professional help arrives.

HEAT CRAMPS

IMPORTANT

- Heat cramps may occur alone or as one of the early symptoms of heat exhaustion or heatstroke; see **HEAT EXHAUSTION** and **HEATSTROKE (SUNSTROKE).**

SYMPTOMS

Sudden onset of severe intermittent muscle pain or spasm following strenuous work or exercise in high heat and humidity. Often affects the calf, thigh or abdomen, but may be felt elsewhere. May include: Pale, moist skin.

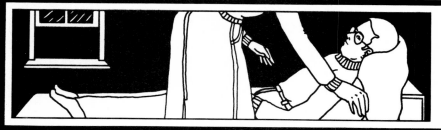

1 Take the person out of the heat to a cool, shaded, well-ventilated area.

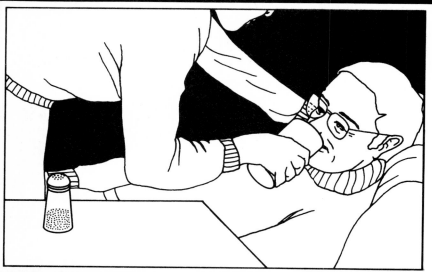

2 Give him sips of salt water (2 pinches of salt in 8 to 10 ounces of water), ½ glass every 15 minutes for about 1 hour. **Do not** use more than the recommended dosage of salt.

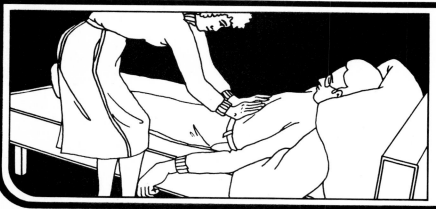

3 To help relieve muscle cramp, apply warm packs and gently massage the affected area or apply pressure with your hands.

HEAT EXHAUSTION

SYMPTOMS

Pale, cold and moist skin. Profuse sweating. Body temperature is about normal. Early symptoms may also include: Muscle cramps. Nausea. Fainting.

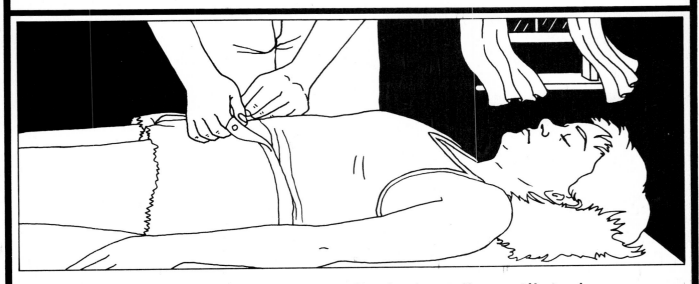

1 Take the person to a cool, shaded, well-ventilated room. Loosen her clothing and have her lie down. Cool her off with fans, an air-conditioner or cool moist cloths.

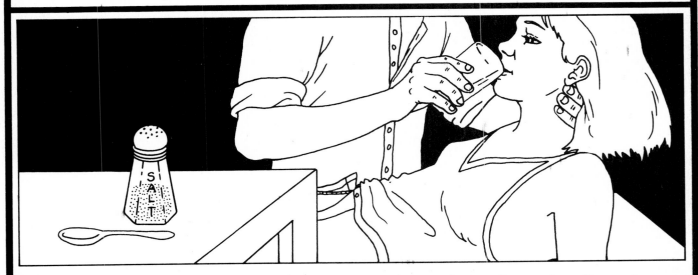

2 If the person is conscious, give her sips of cool salt water (2 pinches of salt in an 8 ounce glass) every few minutes for one hour. Have the person rest, then give her sips of cool water without salt.

HEAT RASH (PRICKLY HEAT)

IMPORTANT

- Consult your doctor if the rash persists or worsens.

- Try to keep the person from scratching at the rash.

- May be prevented by wearing light, loose-fitting clothing made of cotton or other absorbent material.

SYMPTOMS

Burning, prickling sensation around the underarm, thigh or groin. May affect other parts of the body. Sometimes accompanied by itching. Usually occurs in high heat and humidity or when a person is overdressed. Progresses to tiny red and pink pinpoints or blisters. The affected area may become inflamed. Commonly affects infants and overweight adults.

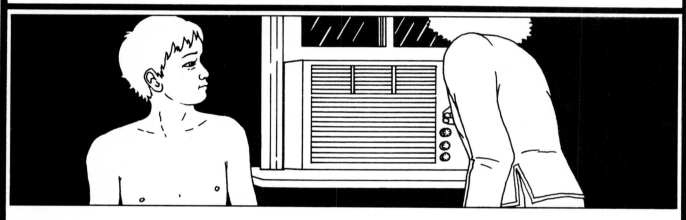

1 Take the person to a cool, shaded, well-ventilated or air-conditioned room.

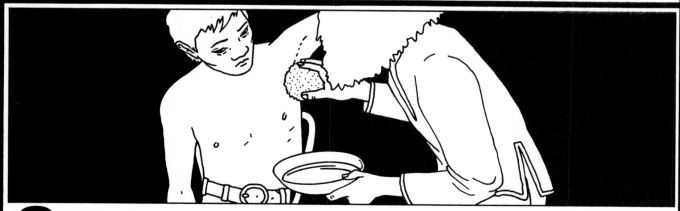

2 Sponge the affected area with cool water. Gently blot dry.

HEAT RASH (PRICKLY HEAT)

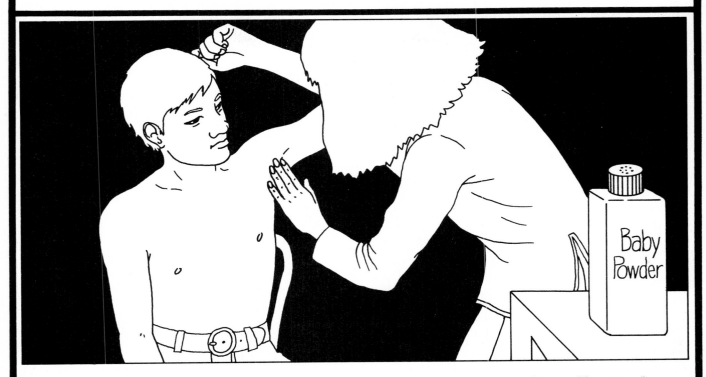

3 Lightly apply baby powder or cornstarch to the affected area to keep it dry.

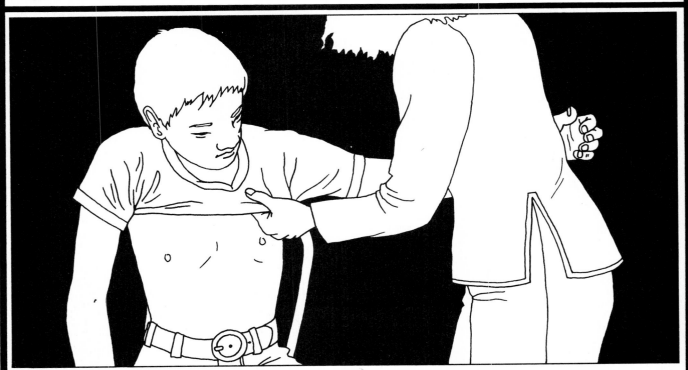

4 Change damp clothing and avoid further sweating.

HEATSTROKE (SUNSTROKE)

IMPORTANT

- **Seek medical aid immediately.**

- Act quickly. Body temperature must be lowered at once. Recheck temperature every 10 minutes. **Do not** reduce temperature below 101°F./38.3°C. Repeat first aid if temperature rises.

- **Do not** give stimulants.

- **Do not** chill.

- Treat for shock; see **SHOCK.**

SYMPTOMS

Body temperature is extremely high (105°F./40.5°C. or higher). Skin is flushed and dry. No sweating. May also include: Muscle cramps. Nausea. Weakness. Collapse. Convulsions. Unconsciousness.

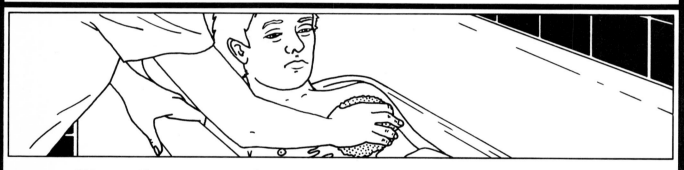

1A Place the person in a partially filled tub of cool water. Using light, brisk strokes, sponge his entire body until the temperature is reduced.

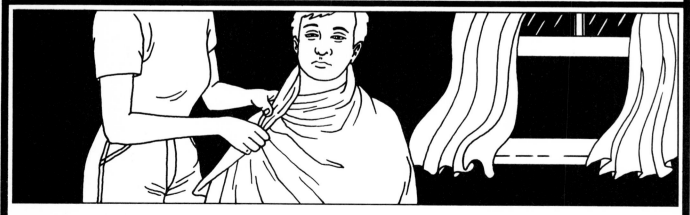

1B Or take the person to a cool well-ventilated room and wrap him in cold wet sheets until temperature is reduced.

HYPOGLYCEMIA (LOW BLOOD SUGAR)

IMPORTANT

- **If the person is unconscious, seek medical aid immediately.**
- Treat for shock; see **SHOCK.**
- **Do not** administer prescribed insulin.
- **Do not** give the person anything to drink if he is unconscious.

SYMPTOMS

May affect anyone, though especially common in diabetics who are reacting to an excessive dose of insulin or who have taken a prescribed dose of insulin, then engaged in excessive exercise or have missed a meal. **Sudden appearance of:** Moist, clammy, ashen or pale skin. Profuse cold sweat. **May include:** Hunger. Shallow breathing. Confusion. Trembling hands. Shaking. Anxiety. Weakness. Dizziness. Personality change. **May progress to:** Convulsions. Coma.

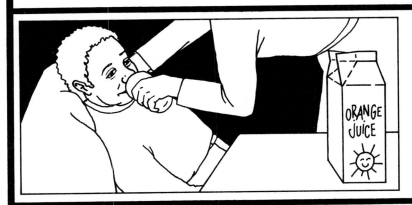

IF THE PERSON IS CONSCIOUS

Give him orange juice, soft drinks containing sugar, candy or sugar in any form.

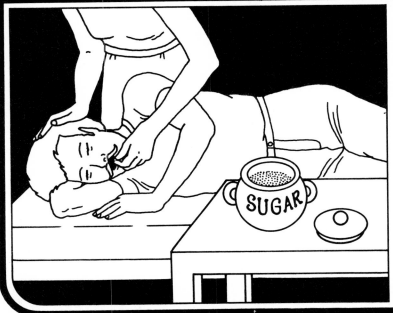

IF THE PERSON IS UNCONSCIOUS

Turn him on his side to keep the airway open and place a pinch of sugar under his tongue. When sugar has dissolved, repeat the dose. Continue small doses of sugar until he regains consciousness.

HYPOTHERMIA

IMPORTANT

- Hypothermia is a life-threatening emergency caused by the severe lowering of the temperature of the core of the body. It is usually caused by cold or cool temperatures, wind, immersion in water or wet clothing. Older persons can also be affected if indoor temperatures are too low, particularly if they are poorly nourished or suffer from chronic illness. Hypothermia may become extremely serious in a matter of minutes or develop slowly over the course of hours or days.

- If symptoms are present, treat for **HYPOTHERMIA** even if the person claims to be fine.

- **Seek medical aid immediately.** A person who has received emergency first aid for hypothermia should be examined by a doctor even if he appears to have recovered fully.

- **Do not** let the person walk or drink anything.

- **Do not** rub the person's body. Handle him very gently. Unnecessary manipulation may cause heart failure.

- Watch breathing closely. If it stops, see **BREATHING: ARTIFICIAL RESPIRATION.**

SYMPTOMS

May or may not show: Persistent or violent shivering. Slow or slurred speech. Personality change. Loss of control over hands. Stumbling. Drowsiness. Impaired reasoning. Confusion. The person may fail to acknowledge symptoms. **In advanced stages:** Muscle spasms and rigidity. Inability to use the arms or legs. Unconsciousness which may mimic death.

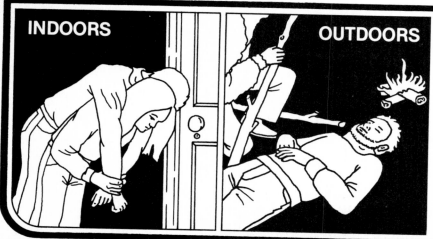

INDOORS OUTDOORS

1 Gently carry the person out of the wind and cold to a warm place, preferably indoors. If that isn't possible, start a fire and improvise a shelter.

HYPOTHERMIA

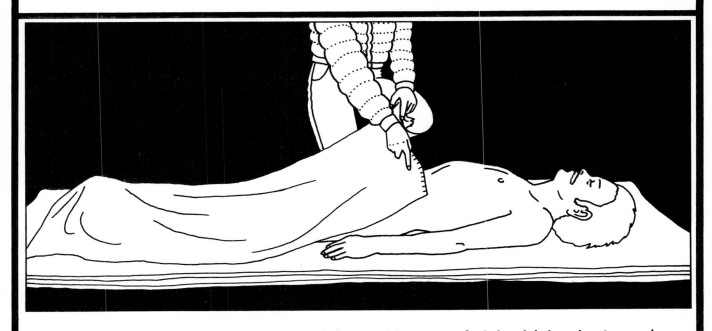

2 Gently remove wet clothing Place a folded blanket under him to insulate him from the cold, and wrap him in a blanket.

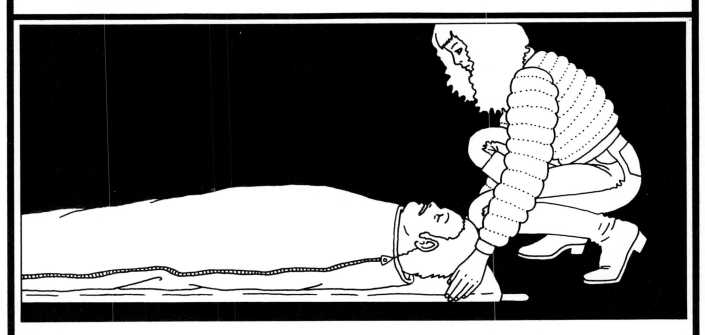

3A **If hypothermia has developed quickly** (as in the case of immersion in cold water): Gently place him in a sleeping bag or several blankets and transport him to medical aid; see **TRANSPORTING THE INJURED.**

CONTINUED ON NEXT PAGE

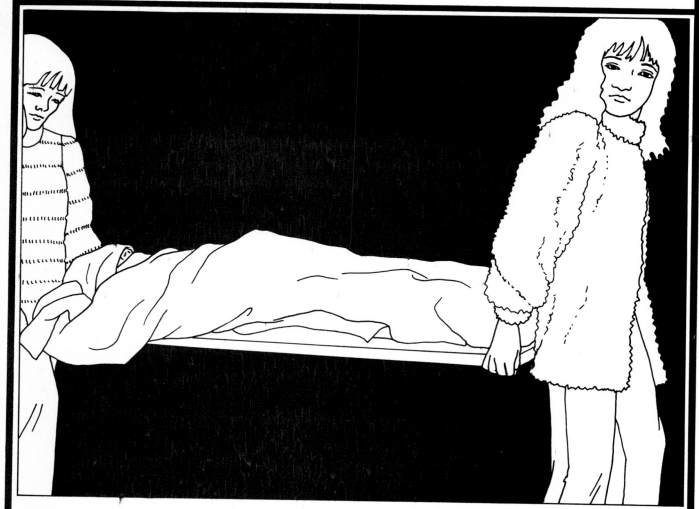

3B **If hypothermia has developed slowly over several hours or days** (as in the case of a lost hunter or an older person in an unheated room): Protect the person from further heat loss by gently wrapping him in a blanket. Loosely cover his head with a scarf or other suitable cloth to conserve heat further and pre-warm the air he breathes. If possible, further insulate the person from wind and cold by placing him in a sleeping bag or wrapping him in a sheet of plastic or plastic garbage bags. Transport him to medical aid, even if it will take hours; see **TRANSPORTING THE INJURED.** If travel is impossible and medical aid cannot reach you, rewarm the person **slowly** by exposing him to warm room air. **Do not** use hot-water bottles, heated towels or any other active rewarming technique.

MOUTH INJURIES

GUMS, PALATE, TEETH, LIPS & TONGUE

IMPORTANT

- Check if there are more serious injuries to the head or neck. If necessary, see **HEAD INJURIES** and **BACK & NECK INJURIES.**

- Clear the mouth of broken teeth. Bring them to the doctor or dentist for possible replanting.

- Lean the person slightly forward so he does not inhale blood.

GUMS & PALATE

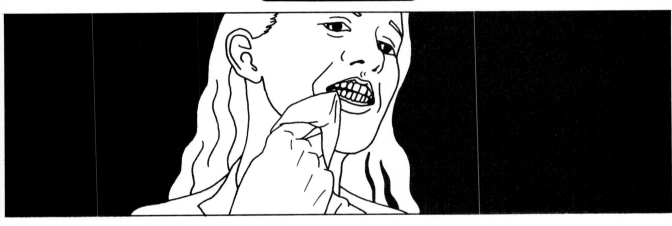

Control bleeding by direct pressure.

TEETH

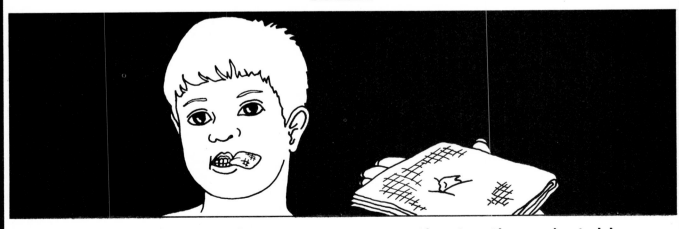

Control bleeding by direct pressure on the tooth socket. Have the person bite down firmly to hold dressing in place.

CONTINUED ON NEXT PAGE

MOUTH INJURIES

GUMS, PALATE, TEETH, LIPS & TONGUE
CONTINUED

LIPS

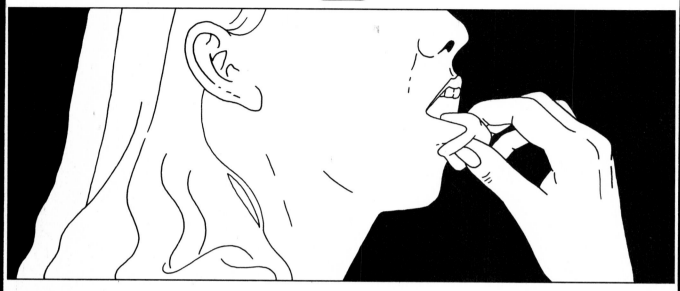

Control bleeding by pressing both sides of the wound.

TONGUE

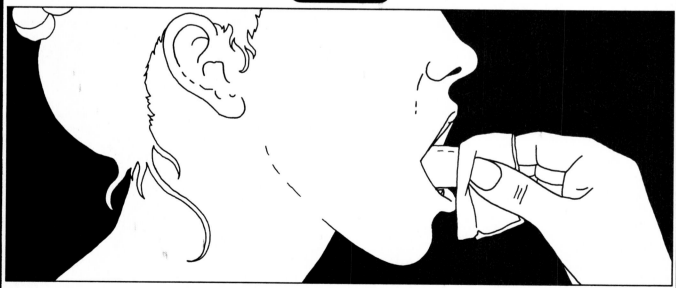

Control bleeding by pressing both sides of the tongue. For more severe bleeding, gently pull the tongue and hold it for about 5 minutes.

MUSCLE CRAMP (CHARLEY HORSE)

IMPORTANT

• Try to relax the affected area. Tension can worsen the muscle spasm.

SYMPTOMS

Sudden spasm and pain in a muscle, usually the calf or thigh. May worsen with movement and limit use of the affected area. Often occurs following overexertion, injury or exposure to cold or dampness. In severe cases, discomfort may last several days or longer.

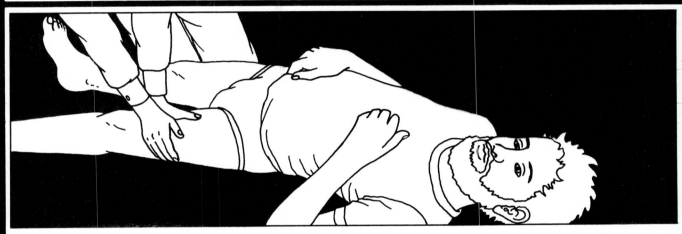

1 Stretch the cramped muscle and apply firm pressure to the affected area with your hands until the cramp is relieved.

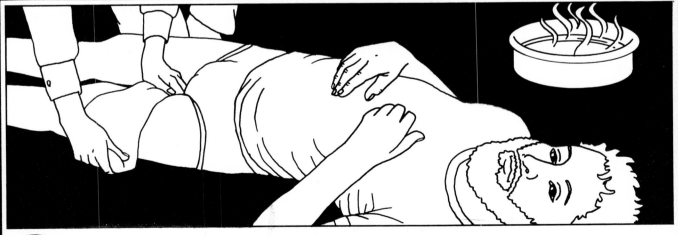

2 Apply warm wet compresses or a hot-water bottle.

3 Have the person rest the affected part.

NOSE INJURIES

BROKEN NOSE, FOREIGN OBJECTS & NOSEBLEED

BROKEN NOSE

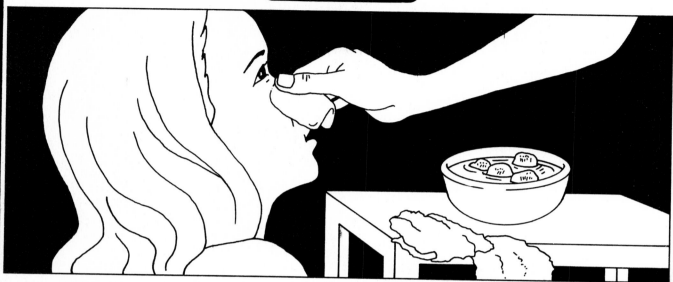

Control the bleeding as for **NOSEBLEED.** Tilt the person's head back slightly, and gently press cold compresses over the nose. **Do not** splint. **Seek medical aid.**

FOREIGN OBJECTS

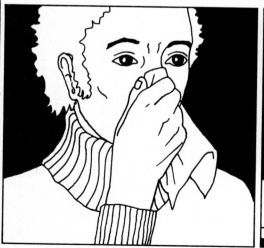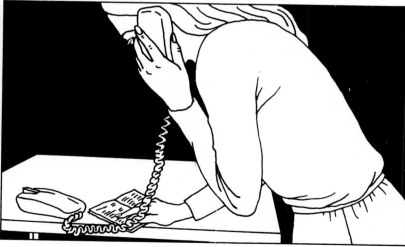

Do not let the person inhale through his nose. Have him blow his nose gently, keeping both nostrils open. **If the object does not come easily, seek medical aid immediately.**

NOSE INJURIES

BROKEN NOSE, FOREIGN OBJECTS & NOSEBLEED

NOSEBLEED

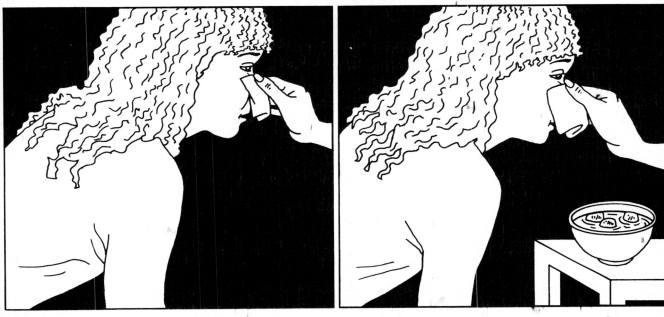

1 Lean the person forward and gently pinch the lower, soft part of the nose for about 5 minutes, then apply cold compresses.

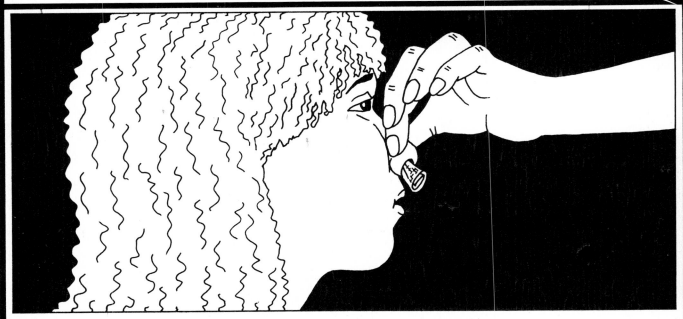

2 If bleeding persists, pack the nostril with gauze, then pinch the nose closed for about 10 minutes.

POISONING

SWALLOWED POISONS

IMPORTANT

- **Call your local Poison Control Center immediately. If you cannot reach the Center, seek other medical aid.**

- Save the poison container and a sample of the vomit.

- Watch breathing closely. If necessary, see **BREATHING: ARTIFICIAL RESPIRATION.**

- **If the person is unconscious, do not** give him anything to drink.

- **Ingredients in products may change over time, and antidotes or counterdoses given on labels may be outdated, obsolete or incorrect. Always consult your local Poison Control Center or other professional medical aid. The following chart and subsequent treatments are to be used only when no emergency medical aid is available.**

If you cannot reach a Poison Control Center or other medical aid:

- Find the poison swallowed on the list on the next page.

- Follow the corresponding treatment on the following pages.

- If you don't know what was swallowed, follow treatment **A**. If there are no burns around the mouth, also have the person drink activated charcoal mixed in a glass of water. Determine the proper dosage by consulting the chart below.

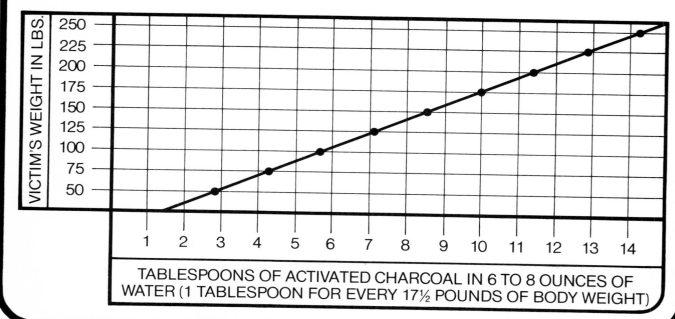

VICTIM'S WEIGHT IN LBS. (250, 225, 200, 175, 150, 125, 100, 75, 50)

TABLESPOONS OF ACTIVATED CHARCOAL IN 6 TO 8 OUNCES OF WATER (1 TABLESPOON FOR EVERY 17½ POUNDS OF BODY WEIGHT)

POISONING

SWALLOWED POISONS

Aspirin or Aspirin Substitutes Ⓑ
Acetone Ⓑ
After Shave Lotion Ⓑ
Alcohol Ⓑ
Antifreeze Ⓑ
Arsenic Ⓑ
Battery Acid Ⓐ
Benzene Ⓑ
Bichloride of Mercury Ⓑ
Bleach Ⓑ
Body Conditioner Ⓑ
Boric Acid Ⓑ
Brush Cleaner Ⓐ
Camphor Ⓑ
Carbon Tetrachloride Ⓑ
Charcoal Lighter Ⓐ
Chlordane Ⓑ
Cologne Ⓑ
Corn Remover Ⓐ
Cosmetics Ⓑ
DDT Ⓑ
Deodorant Ⓑ
Detergent Ⓑ
Dishwasher Granules Ⓐ
Drain Cleaner Ⓐ

Fabric Softeners Ⓑ
Fingernail Polish & Remover Ⓑ
Fireworks Ⓑ
Floor Polish Ⓐ
Flouride Ⓑ
Furniture Polish Ⓐ
Gasoline Ⓐ
Grease Remover Ⓐ
Gun Cleaner Ⓐ
Hair Dye Ⓑ
Hair Permanent Neutralizer Ⓑ
Hair Preparations Ⓑ
Hydrogen Peroxide Ⓑ
Indelible Markers Ⓑ
Ink (Green & Purple) Ⓑ
Insecticides Ⓑ
Iodine Ⓑ
Kerosene Ⓐ
Lacquer Thinner Ⓐ
Liniment Ⓑ
Lye Ⓐ
Matches (more than 20 wooden
      matches or 2 matchbooks) Ⓑ
Mercury Salts Ⓑ
Metal Cleaner Ⓐ

Mothballs, Flakes or Cakes Ⓑ
Naphtha Ⓐ
Oil of Wintergreen Ⓑ
Oven Cleaner Ⓐ
Paint (Lead) Ⓑ
Paint Thinner Ⓐ
Perfume Ⓑ
Pesticides Ⓑ
Pine Oil Ⓑ
Quicklime Ⓐ
Rat or Mouse Poison Ⓑ
Roach Poison Ⓑ
Shoe Polish Ⓐ
Strychnine Ⓑ
Suntan Preparations Ⓑ
Toilet Bowl Cleaner Ⓐ
Turpentine Ⓑ
Typewriter Cleaner Ⓐ
Wart Remover Ⓐ
Washing Soda Ⓐ
Wax (Floor or Furniture) Ⓐ
Weed Killer Ⓐ
Wick Deodorizer Ⓑ
Wood Preservative Ⓐ
Zinc Compounds Ⓐ

 FOR ACID, ALKALI & PETROLEUM POISONING

IMPORTANT

- **Do not induce vomiting.**

SYMPTOMS OF ACID & ALKALI POISONING

Burns around the mouth, lips and tongue. Burning sensations in the mouth, throat and stomach. Cramps. Disorientation. Bloody diarrhea.

SYMPTOMS OF PETROLEUM POISONING

Burning irritation. Coughing. Gagging. Coma. May include petroleum product odor on the breath.

1 If the person is conscious, give him 1 or 2 glasses of milk to dilute the poison. (If milk isn't available, use water.)

2 Loosen tight clothing, then treat for shock; see **SHOCK**.

CONTINUED ON NEXT PAGE

SWALLOWED POISONS
CONTINUED

B **FOR OTHER POISONING**

IMPORTANT

• **Do not** wait for symptoms to develop.

SYMPTOMS

May be intermittent and develop slowly or quickly. May include: Nausea. Dizziness. Drowsiness. Slurred speech. Lack of coordination. Cold clammy skin. Thirst. Convulsions. Coma.

1 If the person is conscious, give him 1 or 2 glasses of water to dilute the poison.

2 If he has not vomited, induce vomiting by giving him syrup of ipecac (2 tablespoons for an adult, 1 tablespoon for a child over 1 year of age, 2 teaspoons for an infant) followed by a glass of water. Keep the person moving. If he doesn't vomit within 30 minutes, give him a second dose followed by another glass of water, but **do not** repeat a third time. If he still hasn't vomited within the next 30 minutes, try to induce vomiting by placing your finger on the back of his tongue. **Use this method immediately if ipecac isn't available.**

3 When he starts to vomit, make sure his head is between his legs. Hold a small child face down over your knee.

4 When he has finished vomiting, have the person drink activated charcoal mixed in a glass of water. Determine the proper dosage by consulting the chart below.

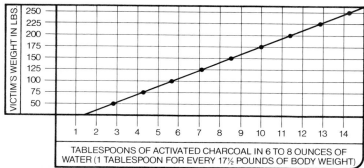

TABLESPOONS OF ACTIVATED CHARCOAL IN 6 TO 8 OUNCES OF WATER (1 TABLESPOON FOR EVERY 17½ POUNDS OF BODY WEIGHT)

5 Loosen tight clothing and treat for shock; see **SHOCK.**

POISONING

INHALED POISONS

IMPORTANT

- **Seek medical aid and oxygen immediately.**

- **Also call your local Poison Control Center.**

- Watch breathing closely. If necessary, see **BREATHING: ARTIFICIAL RESPIRATION.**

SYMPTOMS

Irritated eyes, nose, throat or lungs. Coughing. Headache. Shortness of breath. Nausea. Dizziness. Convulsions. Unconsciousness. Caused by auto exhaust or chemical fumes from paints, solvents and industrial gases.

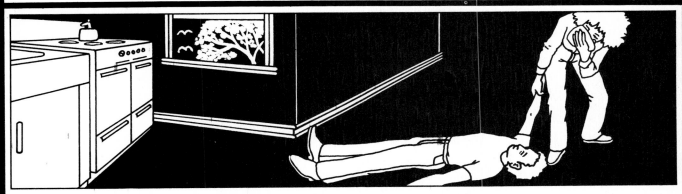

1 Remove the person from the source of the poison. Be careful not to inhale the poison yourself.

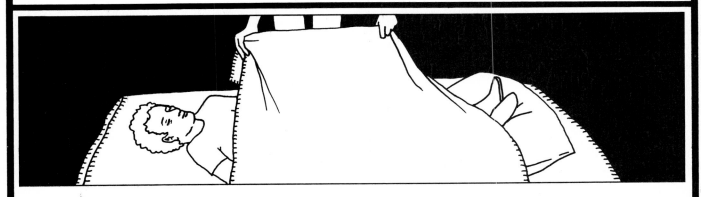

2 Loosen tight clothing and treat for shock; see **SHOCK.** Keep him from becoming chilled. If his skin is affected by chemical vapor or mist, see **BURNS: CHEMICAL.**

CONTACT

IMPORTANT

- **Seek medical aid if there is a severe reaction or the person is highly allergic.**

- Watch breathing closely. If necessary, see **BREATHING: ARTIFICIAL RESPIRATION.**

- Treat for shock; see **SHOCK.**

SYMPTOMS

Burning and itching. Rash. Blisters. Swelling. Headache. Fever.

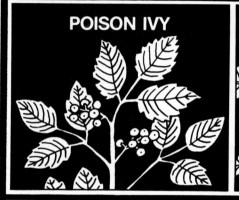

POISON IVY

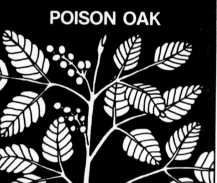

POISON OAK

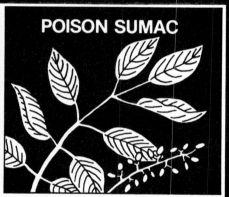

POISON SUMAC

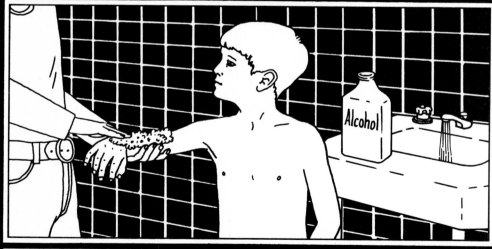

1 Remove contaminated clothing. Wash all affected areas thoroughly with soap and water, then apply rubbing alcohol.

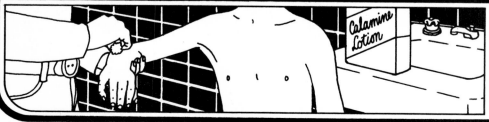

2 Apply calamine lotion to ease the itching.

POISONING: PLANTS

INGESTED

IMPORTANT

- **Call your local Poison Control Center immediately. Also seek medical aid.**

- Watch breathing closely. If necessary, see **BREATHING: ARTIFICIAL RESPIRATION.**

- **If the person is unconscious, do not** give him anything to drink.

- **If you cannot reach a Poison Control Center or medical aid, see POISONING (SWALLOWED POISONS),** and follow treatment **B.**

BANEBERRY

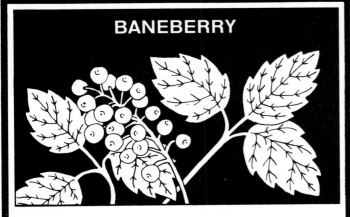

SYMPTOMS
Dizziness. Cramps. Vomiting. Headache. Delirium.

BITTERSWEET

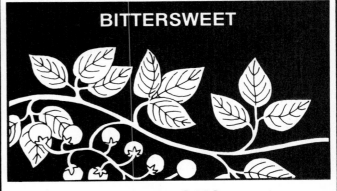

SYMPTOMS
Burning sensation in the throat. Nausea. Dizziness. Dilated pupils. Weakness. Convulsions.

CASTOR BEAN

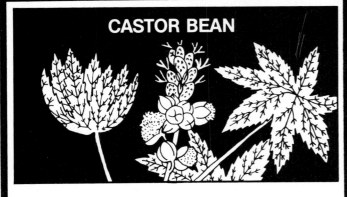

SYMPTOMS
Burning sensations in the mouth and throat. Nausea. Vomiting. Cramps. Stupor. Convulsions.

DAPHNE

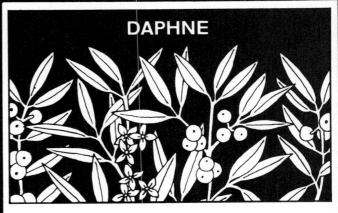

SYMPTOMS
Burning sensations in the mouth, throat and stomach. Cramps.

CONTINUED ON NEXT PAGE

INGESTED
CONTINUED

FOXGLOVE

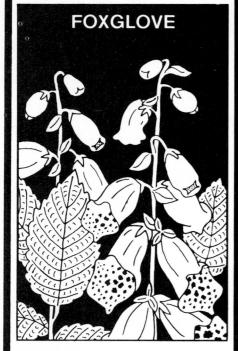

SYMPTOMS
Nausea. Upset stomach. Dizziness. Disorientation.

JIMSON WEED

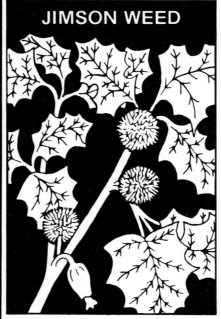

SYMPTOMS
Extreme thirst. Impaired vision. Rapid heartbeat. Dilated pupils. Delirium. Coma.

LARKSPUR

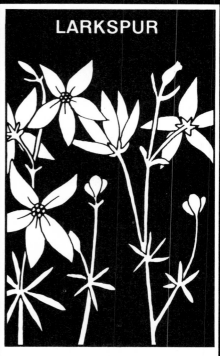

SYMPTOMS
Tingling in the mouth. Upset stomach. Anxiety. Severe depression.

LILY-OF-THE-VALLEY

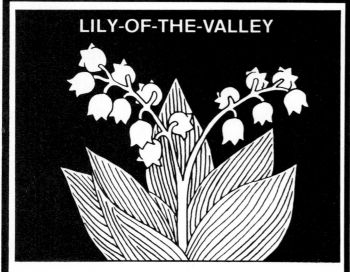

SYMPTOMS
Upset stomach. Dizziness. Vomiting. Disorientation.

MONKSHOOD

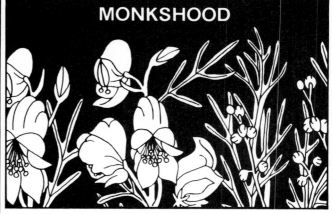

SYMPTOMS
Tingling or numbness of the lips and tongue. Excessive salivation. Dizziness. Nausea. Vomiting. Dimmed vision.

INGESTED

NIGHTSHADE

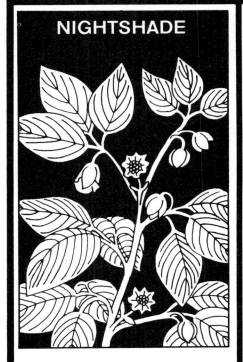

SYMPTOMS
Thirst. Upset stomach. Numbness. Rapid heart-beat.

POISON HEMLOCK

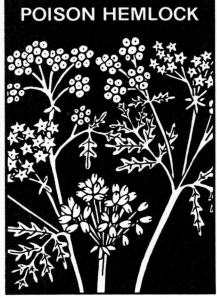

SYMPTOMS
Burning sensations in the mouth and throat. Weakness. Paralysis of the arms and chest. Stupor.

POKEWEED

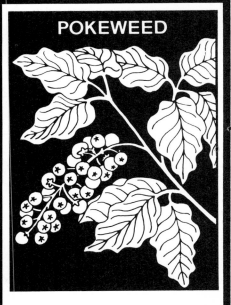

SYMPTOMS
Burning sensations in the mouth and throat. Nausea. Cramps. Upset stomach. Vomiting. Drowsiness. Impaired vision.

WATER HEMLOCK

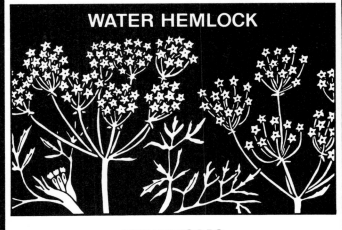

SYMPTOMS
Excessive salivation. Foaming at the mouth. Stomach pain. Frenzy. Shivering. Irregular breathing. Delirium. Violent convulsions.

YEW

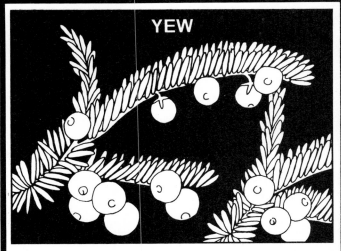

SYMPTOMS
Nausea. Stomach pain. Vomiting. Shivering. Difficulty breathing. Diarrhea.

MUSHROOM POISONING

IMPORTANT

- Call your local Poison Control Center immediately if you know or suspect that a poisonous mushroom has been ingested. Also seek medical aid.

- **If you cannot reach a Poison Control Center or medical aid,** begin treatment immediately. **Do not** wait for symptoms to develop.

- Save a sample of the vomit and, if possible, the mushroom.

- **Do not** give the person anything alcoholic to drink.

- **If he is unconscious, do not** give him **anything** to drink.

SYMPTOMS

Depending on the mushroom, symptoms may develop rapidly (from minutes to about 2 hours) or slowly (from 6 to 24 hours). **May include:** Profuse salivation or drooling. Tearing of the eyes. Headache. Nausea. Sweating. Tiny pupils. Vomiting. Stomach cramps. Severe diarrhea. Dizziness and confusion. Coma. **In delayed reactions, symptoms may also include:** Passage of little or no urine. After 2 to 3 days, jaundiced (yellowed) skin and eyes.

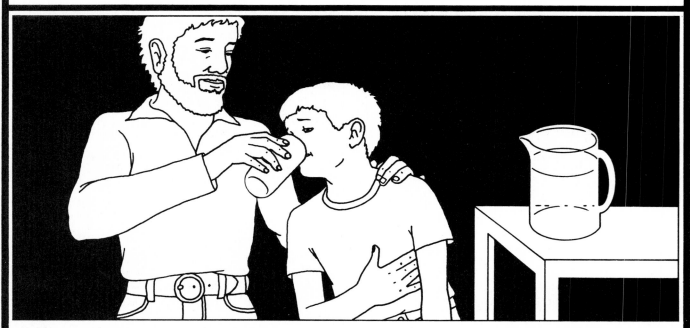

1 If the person is conscious, give him 1 or 2 glasses of water or milk to dilute the poison.

MUSHROOM POISONING

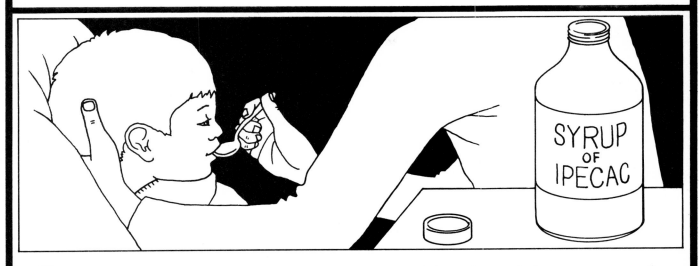

2 If he has not vomited, induce vomiting by giving syrup of ipecac (2 tablespoons for an adult, 1 tablespoon for a child over 1 year of age, 2 teaspoons for an infant), followed by a glass of water. Keep the person moving. If he doesn't vomit within 30 minutes, give him a second dose followed by another glass of water, but **do not** repeat a third time. If he still hasn't vomited within the next 30 minutes, try to induce vomiting by placing your finger on the back of his tongue. **Use this method immediately if ipecac isn't available.**

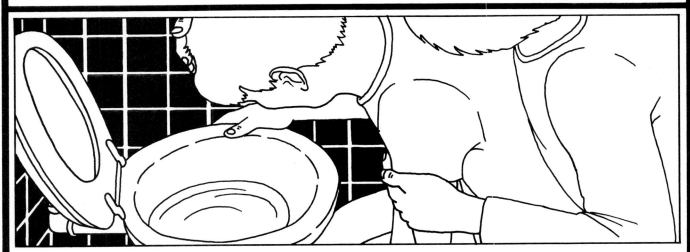

3 When he starts to vomit, make sure his head is between his legs. Hold a small child face down over your knee.

CONTINUED ON NEXT PAGE

MUSHROOM POISONING
CONTINUED

4 When he has finished vomiting, have the person drink activated charcoal mixed in a glass of water. Determine the proper dosage by consulting the chart below.

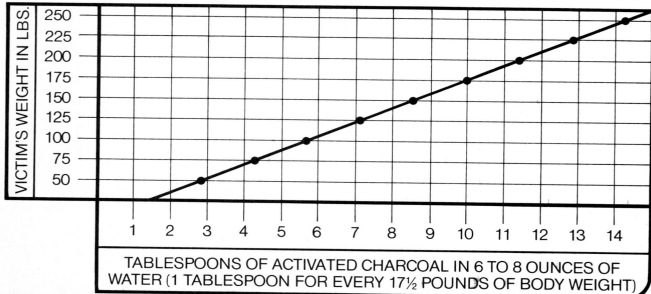

VICTIM'S WEIGHT IN LBS.

TABLESPOONS OF ACTIVATED CHARCOAL IN 6 TO 8 OUNCES OF WATER (1 TABLESPOON FOR EVERY 17½ POUNDS OF BODY WEIGHT)

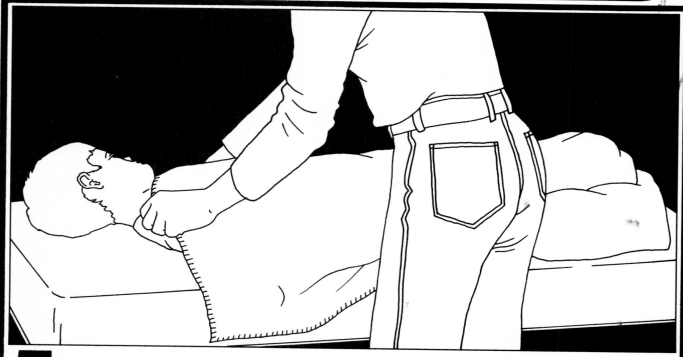

5 Loosen tight clothing and treat for shock; see **SHOCK.**

SHOCK

- **Always treat a seriously injured person for shock.**
- **Do not** give him anything to drink.
- **Do not** overheat.
- **Seek medical aid immediately.**

SYMPTOMS

Pale or bluish lips, gums, skin and fingernails. Clammy skin, mottled in color. Weakness. Breathing is weak and shallow or deep but irregular. May also include: Anxiety. Apathy. Nausea. Thirst.

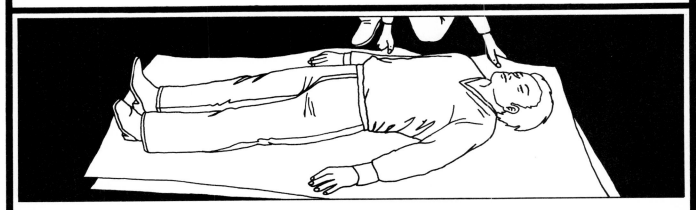

1 Lay the person down. Place a blanket under him if he is cold or damp, but **do not** move him if his back or neck is injured.

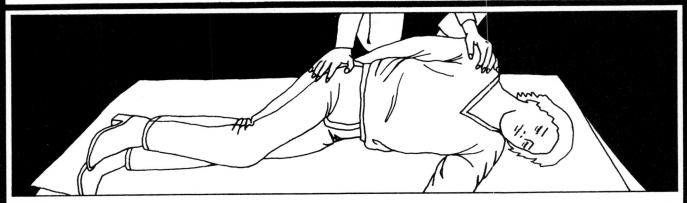

2A If he has no back or neck injuries and is unconscious or bleeding heavily from the jaw or lower face, turn him on his side to keep the airway open. In the case of an open chest injury, turn him onto the injured side.

CONTINUED ON NEXT PAGE

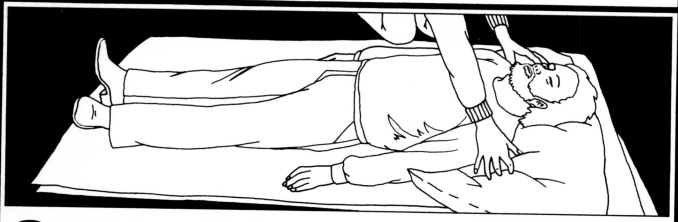

2B If he has no back or neck injuries and his head is injured or he has trouble breathing, elevate his head and shoulders.

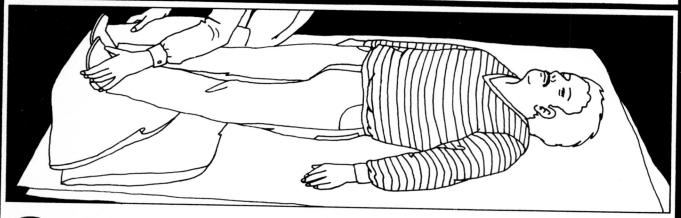

2C Otherwise, elevate his legs about 8 to 12 inches, unless that causes pain.

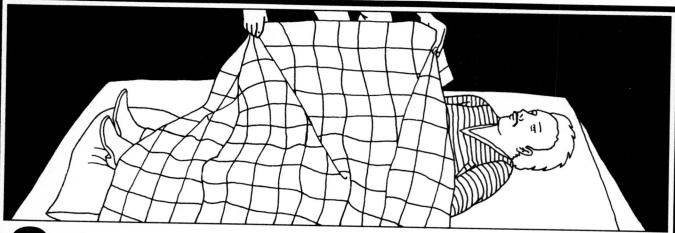

3 Cover him lightly with a blanket to prevent loss of body heat.

SPLINTERS

IMPORTANT

- **Seek medical aid** if the splinter is deeply embedded beneath the skin or if signs of infection develop after it has been removed.
- Wash your hands thoroughly before you attempt to remove the splinter.

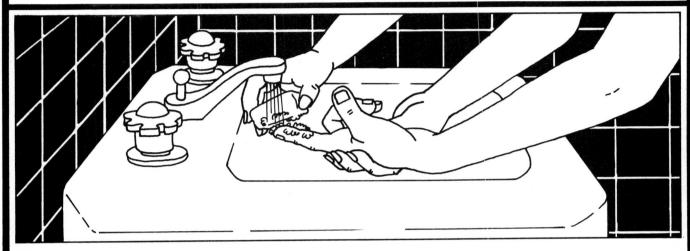

1 Gently wash the area around the splinter with soap and water.

IF THE SPLINTER IS PROTRUDING FROM THE SKIN

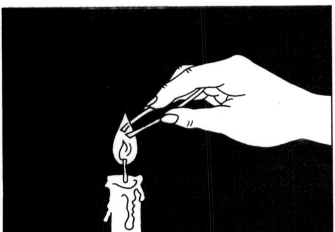 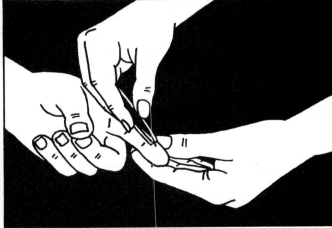

2A Sterilize a tweezers by holding it over an open flame or soaking it for ten minutes in rubbing alcohol or boiling water, then gently remove the splinter at the same angle at which it entered.

CONTINUED ON NEXT PAGE

159

SPLINTERS

IF THE SPLINTER IS EMBEDDED JUST UNDER THE SKIN

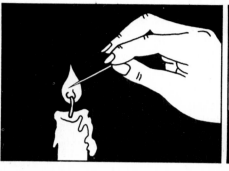 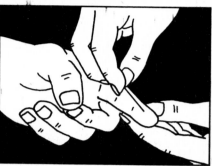 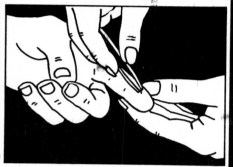

2B Sterilize a needle by holding it over an open flame or soaking it for ten minutes in rubbing alcohol or boiling water, then gently loosen the skin around the splinter and remove it with a sterilized tweezers at the same angle at which it entered.

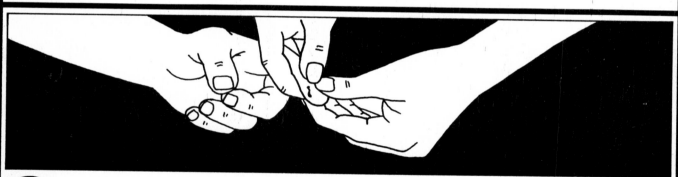

3 Squeeze the wound gently so that it bleeds slightly.

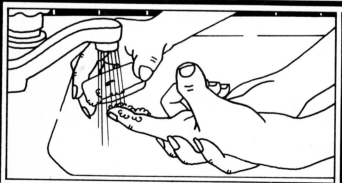 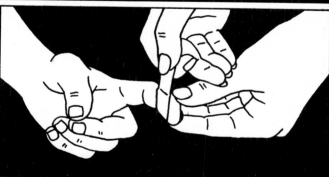

4 Wash the affected area with soap and water, then cover with a bandage.

SPRAINS & STRAINS

- Keep the person off the injured parts.
- **Do not** pack in ice or immerse in ice water.

SPRAINS

SYMPTOMS

Pain, rapid swelling, tenderness and discoloration of the soft tissue surrounding a joint.

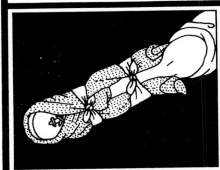 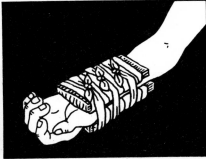

1 Immobilize the injured area with a blanket, splint, pillow, etc. **Do not** bandage too tightly; sprains swell.

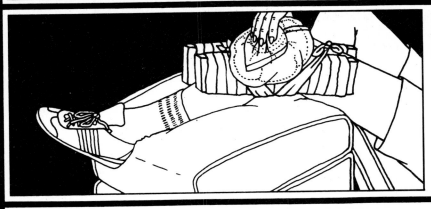

2 To minimize swelling, elevate sprained elbows, knees or ankles. Apply cold, wet compresses or an ice bag covered with a towel.

STRAINS

SYMPTOMS

Pain caused by stretched or pulled muscles.

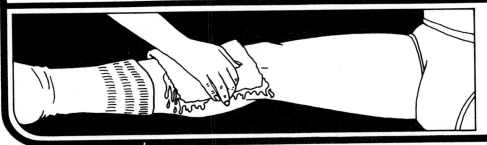

Apply warm, wet compresses and rest the injured part.

STOMACH INJURIES

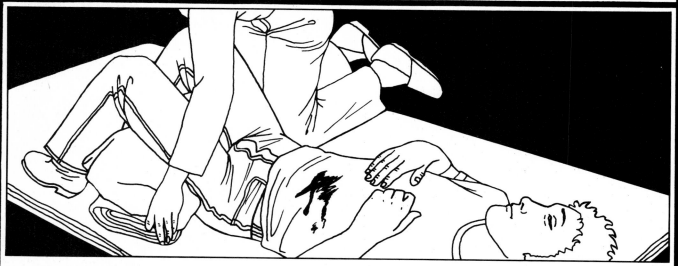

1 Relax the stomach muscles by placing the person on his back with a pillow or blanket under his knees.

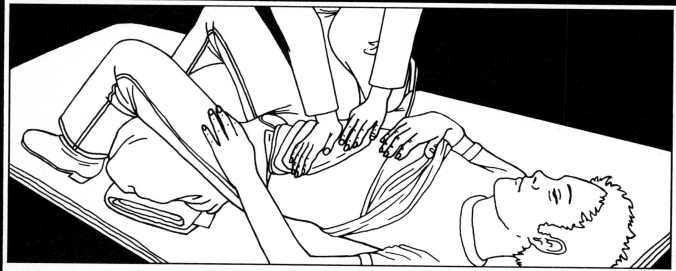

2 Control bleeding by gently applying direct pressure on the wound with gauze or a clean cloth.

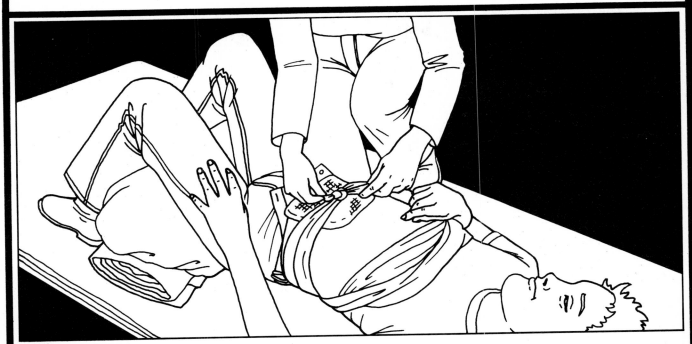

3 Bandage the dressing firmly in place.

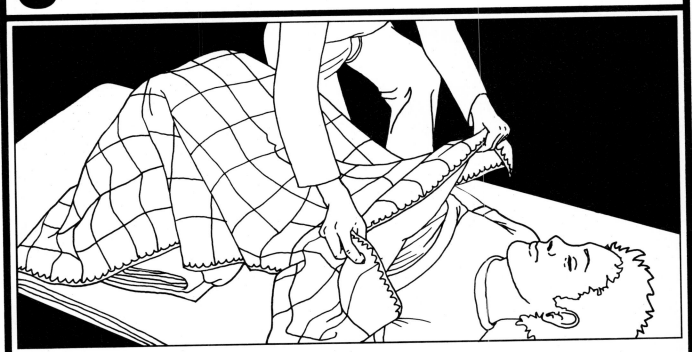

4 If organs or intestines protrude, **do not** attempt to replace them. Cover the area with a clean dressing dampened with sterile or cooled boiled water. Bandage in place firmly but not too tightly. Treat for shock; see **SHOCK**.

TAKING THE PULSE

- In a serious emergency it may be necessary to check the victim's pulse to determine whether the heart has stopped beating and emergency first aid for heart failure should therefore begin. In this case, it is extremely important to find the pulse if one is present since first aid for heart failure is potentially dangerous and should never be performed needlessly. **Do not** rush. Check the pulse slowly and carefully, taking between 5 and 10 seconds to find it.

- **Do not** use your thumb to check the pulse since its own pulse may be mistaken for that of the other person.

- If possible, check the pulse when the person is at rest. The pulse is normally strong and regular. The rate typically rises to reflect increases in activity, body temperature, anxiety, etc. Illness or injury may produce a pulse that is irregular, slow and/or weak.

NORMAL PULSE RATES (AT REST)

Infants & Childen: 90 to 130 beats a minute
Adults: 60 to 100 beats a minute

INFANTS

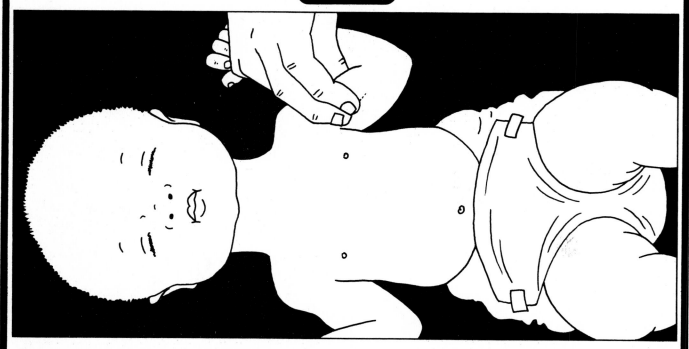

Place the tips of your fingers on the inside of the upper arm.

TAKING THE PULSE

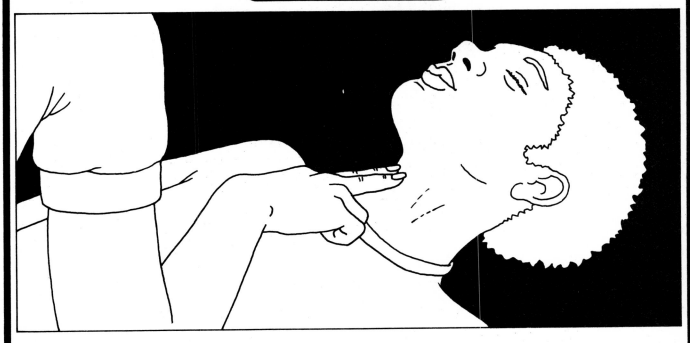

1 Place your first two fingers on the person's Adam's apple (about halfway between the chin and the collarbone).

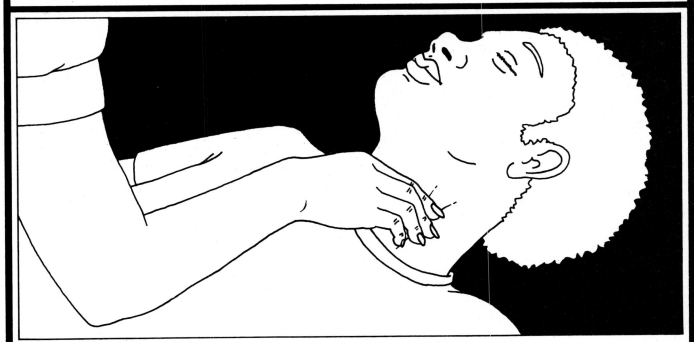

2 Slide your fingers into the groove next to the windpipe on the side nearest you, then press gently.

165

NECK & SPINE INJURIES

IMPORTANT

- **If the person is seriously injured, call an ambulance immediately. Do not move him unless it is a matter of life or death and no ambulance is available.** It is almost always better to wait for proper equipment and expert help. If you must transport the person, get as much aid as possible.

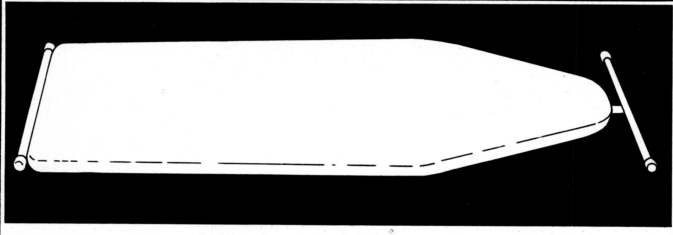

1 Devise a stretcher out of a sturdy board, door, ironing board, etc.

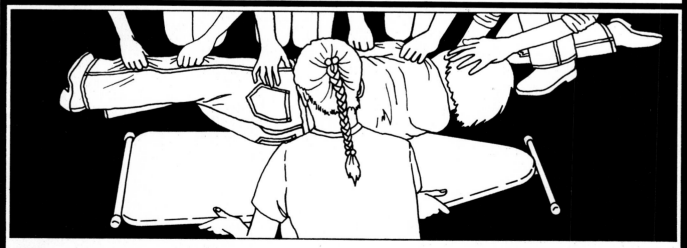

2 **Do not** twist the injured person. Move his body as a single unit, keeping his head in line with his spinal column. On a signal from the person holding the head, roll him gently onto his side and place the stretcher next to him.

NECK & SPINE INJURIES

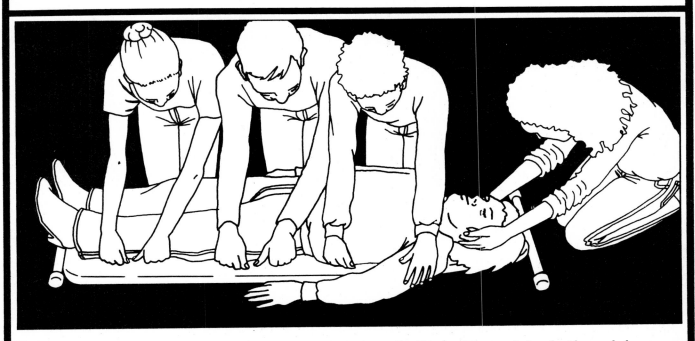

3 Roll him onto the stretcher carefully without twisting his body or head.

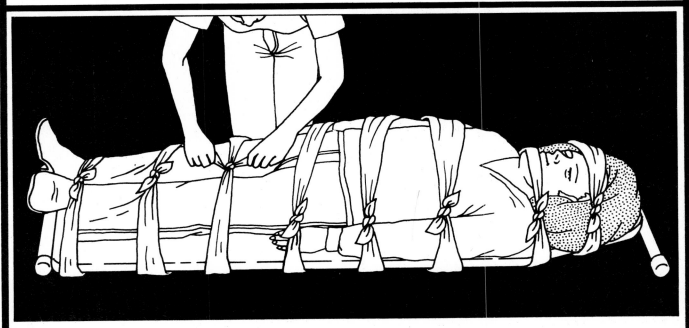

4 Immobilize his head with a rolled blanket or the like. (For spine injuries, also immobilize his torso.) Bind him to the stretcher with bandages, belts, etc.

STRETCHERS & CARRIES

IMPROVISED STRETCHERS

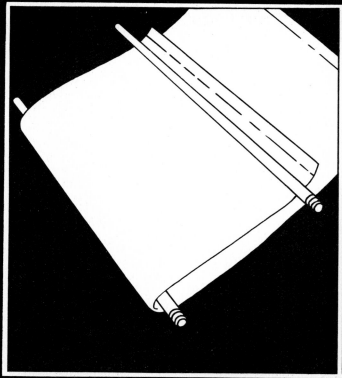
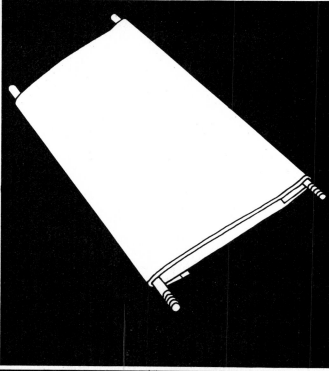
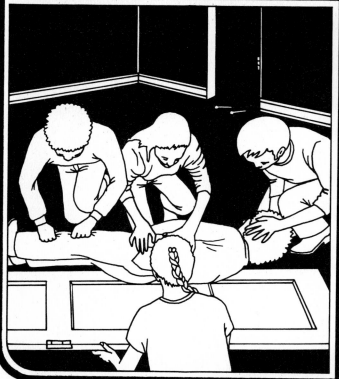
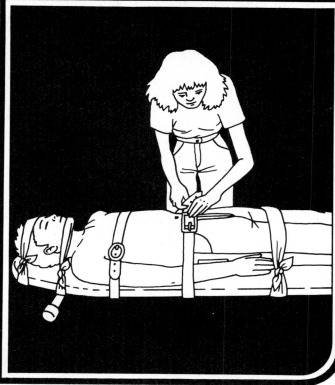

168

TRANSPORTING THE INJURED

STRETCHERS & CARRIES

CARRIES

CHAIR CARRY

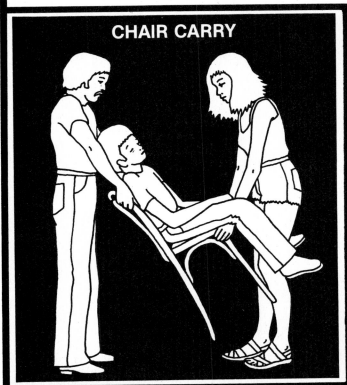

FIREMAN & PACK-STRAP

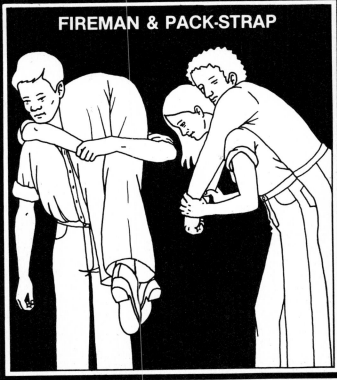

ONE-PERSON LIFT

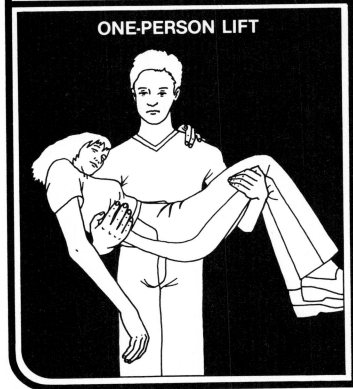

TWO-MAN SEAT

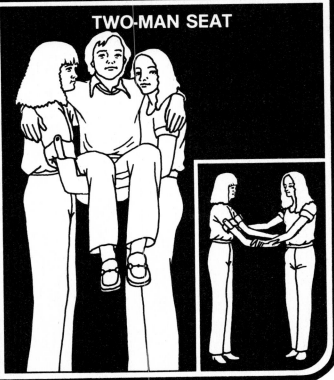

UNCONSCIOUSNESS

IMPORTANT

- **Seek medical aid immediately** if the person does not revive when you call him loudly, tap him on the shoulder or shake him gently. Note how long he remains unconscious and any changes in his state.

- Watch breathing closely. If necessary, see **BREATHING: ARTIFICIAL RESPIRATION.**

- **Do not** move the person unless absolutely necessary. You may cause further harm. If necessary, see **TRANSPORTING THE INJURED.**

- **Do not** give him anything to drink.

- If the cause of unconsciousness is not known, check for signs of injury, hidden bleeding, bites or stings, poisons, drugs, etc. Look for emergency medical information tags around the neck or wrist, or a card in the wallet identifying the possible cause. On hot days or following vigorous exercise, the person may be suffering heat-stroke or heat exhaustion; see **HEATSTROKE (SUNSTROKE)** and **HEAT EXHAUSTION.**

SYMPTOMS

Can vary from a very brief loss of consciousness, from which the person can be easily roused, to a deep coma. Depending on the cause, the face, gums or inner linings of the eyelids may appear either flushed, white or blue.

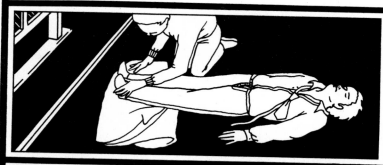

1 Keep the person lying down. Loosen restrictive clothing. Provide good ventilation. Elevate his legs 8 to 12 inches.

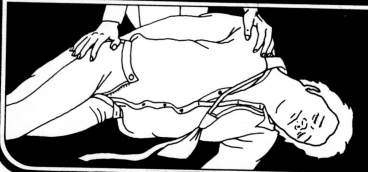

2 If the person vomits, turn his head to the side or roll him onto his side to keep the airway open and allow fluids to drain.

PART TWO

ILLNESSES & DISORDERS

This section describes all the most common illnesses and disorders. It is designed as a reference guide to help you understand and cope with conditions that may impair your family's normal good health. It is not a substitute for professional medical care.

Each illness and disorder is discussed in terms of its common symptoms, underlying causes and, most importantly, what you should do about it. Special precautions and recommendations for prevention are indicated wherever they are appropriate. For infectious diseases, you will also find information about incubation, communicability and duration.

Keep in mind that a person afflicted with a particular ailment may show some, all or none of the listed symptoms. Remember, too, that a given symptom can have any number of causes. Rarely is a symptom so unique that it is seen in one and only one illness.

As a general rule, it is probably best to consult your physician whenever you discover any symptoms of ill health in a family member, even if you are uncertain about them or they seem mild or appear only occasionally. Depending on the cause, some symptoms come on suddenly and are entirely obvious, but others may develop slowly and subtly and be only intermittent. Nor does the apparent severity of the symptom necessarily signify the seriousness of the underlying cause. Minor disorders sometimes produce dramatic symptoms, while far more serious illnesses may have symptoms that are scarcely evident. Your physician would certainly prefer a false alarm to the unnecessary delay that may lead to complications or permit the disorder to worsen.

We have indicated the treatments a physician is likely to prescribe only to give you some idea of what you might expect. Other treatments do exist, as do alternate medical approaches. Although we have noted where surgery is usually employed, should it be recommended, it is advisable to obtain a second opinion.

ALLERGIES

ALLERGIC DRUG REACTIONS

SYMPTOMS

Hives or other skin rash. Unexpected fever. Asthma or hay fever-like reaction. Sometimes: serum sickness; see SERUM SICKNESS. Most feared reaction: anaphylactic shock; see ANAPHYLACTIC SHOCK. Almost any medication, even aspirin, can cause mild or severe allergic reactions in some people. Common causes include penicillin and other antibiotics, local anesthetics, insulin, some tranquilizers.

WHAT TO DO

• **Stop all medication.**
• **Consult your physician.**
• **If the reaction is severe, get to an emergency room at once. Immediate treatment is essential.** May include injections of Adrenalin.
• For home care of milder reactions such as itching, your physician may recommend an oral antihistamine. Compresses dipped in cold milk are often helpful.

ANAPHYLACTIC SHOCK
(Hypersensitivity to insect stings or medications)

SYMPTOMS

Within 15 minutes after a sting from a honeybee, wasp, yellow jacket or hornet or exposure to other sensitizing material: Flushed skin. Agitation. Giant hives. Breathing difficulty. Itching. Coughing. Sneez- ing. May be followed by signs of shock: Pale, cold and clammy skin. Sweaty forehead and palms. Rapid and weak pulse.

WHAT TO DO

• **THIS IS A LIFE-AND-DEATH EMERGENCY. Death can occur in minutes. Get to an emergency room or other medical help immediately.** On the way, apply ice or cold compresses to the sting site. Also try to slow the spread of venom by wrapping a tourniquet above the site. Improvise the tourniquet out of a folded handkerchief, etc. Be sure to loosen the tourniquet every 4 minutes. If caused by a beesting, remove the stinger and venom sac; see **BITES & STINGS: INSECTS** in Part One.
• If prepared with a sting kit — it should be prescribed for and carried by anyone sensitive to insect stings — follow the directions immediately. Get to medical help.

SERUM SICKNESS

SYMPTOMS

Hives or other skin rash. Fever. Joint pains. Lymph node swelling. A delayed allergic reaction that appears 7 to 12 days after administration of an animal serum or, more commonly, penicillin or other drugs to which there is individual sensitivity.

WHAT TO DO

• **Consult your physician.**
• Sickness is self-limiting. Medication may be prescribed to relieve the itching and joint pains.

BLOOD & LYMPH DISORDERS

ANEMIA FROM IRON DEFICIENCY

SYMPTOMS

IN MILD CASES: Lack of energy. Easy fatigability. IN MORE SEVERE CASES: Shortness of breath. Heart pounding. Rapid pulse. IN VERY SEVERE CASES: Weakness. Headache. Dizziness. Drowsiness. Ringing in the ears. Irritability. Spots before the eyes. Stomach and intestinal complaints. Menses failure. Libido loss. Low-grade fever. Psychotic behavior. Caused by a shortage of iron, need to make hemoglobin, the red blood cell pigment that carries oxygen from the lungs to the tissues. May result from inadequate iron in the diet or from chronic **blood loss** through excessive menstruation, a slow-bleeding ulcer, hemorrhoids, gastrointestinal tumors or hookworm.

WHAT TO DO

• **Consult your physician.** May require making certain that iron deficiency is present and not another type of anemia with similar symptoms. The cause might also be chronic blood loss.
• Iron may be prescribed in oral tablet form or, if not well tolerated, by injection. Instead of, or in addition to, the iron, an iron-rich diet may be prescribed that includes such foods as meat (especially liver), eggs, raisins, spinach, whole wheat bread and beet greens.
• Consulting a nutritionist can be helpful.

APLASTIC ANEMIA

SYMPTOMS

May include any or many of the symptoms for iron deficiency anemia (see ANEMIA FROM IRON DEFICIENCY), but are usually more severe. Also may include: Brown skin pigmentation. Blood seeping into the skin. Severe sore throat. Reduced resistance to infections. Results from damage to the bone marrow, where both red and white blood cells are produced (the red needed for tissue nutrition, the white to fight infections). Marrow damage may be caused by some drugs or chemicals such as chloramphenicol, gold compounds, some sulfa drugs, phenylbutazone, quinacrine, methotrexate, nitrogen mustard, benzene and insecticides.

WHAT TO DO

- **Consult your physician.**
- Exposure to the cause must be stopped.
- Treatment may require blood transfusion until the bone marrow can be restored to health. Other measures may include infection control with antibiotics.

HEMOLYTIC ANEMIA

SYMPTOMS

May include any or many of the symptoms for iron deficiency anemia (see ANEMIA FROM IRON DEFICIENCY), but also with some degree of jaundice (skin yellowing). Sometimes includes: Chills. Fever. Nausea. Vomiting. Abdominal pain. Results from red blood cells being destroyed faster than new ones can form. Possible causes include Rh incompatibility, mismatched blood transfusions, industrial poisons such as benzene, trinitrotoluene and aniline, and reactions to some medications.

WHAT TO DO

- **Consult your physician**
- Prompt hospitalization is usually needed for blood transfusion and other treatment.

HEMOPHILIA (Bleeding disease)

SYMPTOMS

Excessive bleeding from minor cuts or wounds. Often includes spontaneous bleeding under the skin and in the gums, gastrointestinal tract, joints and muscles. Bleeding in the joints and muscles sometimes produces joint stiffening. An inherited disorder transmitted only to males by females. Involves an impaired ability of the blood to clot due to deficiency of a blood substance, factor VIII, needed for coagulation.

WHAT TO DO

- **Consult your physician.**
- Treatment requires replacement of the missing blood factor. Serious bleeding episodes may call for blood transfusion.
- A hemophiliac should carry a wallet card or other notice of the disorder to help assure proper treatment in case of an accident.

LYMPHADENITIS

SYMPTOMS

Englargment of one or more lymph nodes (sometimes mistakenly referred to as lymph glands) such as those in the neck, underarms and groin. Accompanied by tenderness and pain. The overlying skin is red and tender and sometimes abscessed. An inflammatory lymph node reaction which can be due to any bacterial, viral or other infectious agent but most often strep and staph bacteria. Can be due to primary infection elsewhere such as in a tooth or finger.

WHAT TO DO

- **Consult your physician.**
- Treatment may require antibiotics; either hot, wet applications or ice packs to relieve pain; incision and drainage of abscesses.

LYMPHANGITIS

SYMPTOMS

Fever (102° to 105°F. / 38.9° to 40.5°C.). Chills. Malaise. Generalized aching. Headache. Lymph node swelling. An inflammation of the lymph channels usually caused by strep or staph bacteria. May spread from infection in a hand or foot, with irregular pink, tender streaks extending up the limb to lymph nodes in the underarm or groin.

WHAT TO DO

- **Consult your physician.**
- Care of the original infection is vital. Suitable antibiotic therapy is usually prescribed. For severe cases, bed rest and elevation of the affected part are required.

PERNICIOUS ANEMIA

SYMPTOMS

May include any or many of the symptoms for iron deficiency anemia (see ANEMIA FROM IRON DEFICIENCY), but also with: Red, sore tongue. Swallowing difficulty. Weight loss. Intermittent constipation. Intermittent diarrhea. Ill-defined abdominal pain. Sometimes: Numbness and tingling of the legs and fingers. Unsteady gait. Irritability. Mild depression. Fever. Caused by inadequate amounts of a substance — intrinsic factor — produced in the stomach and needed for absorption of vitamin B_{12}, which is required for red blood cell production in the bone marrow.

WHAT TO DO

- **Consult your physician.**
- Although vitamin B_{12} cannot be absorbed properly from food or vitamin supplements taken by mouth, injections of B_{12} can bring dramatic improvement.

POLYCYTHEMIA VERA

SYMPTOMS

Often begin with: Easy fatigability. Difficulty concentrating. Headache. Drowsiness. Forgetfulness. Dizziness. Other symptoms may include: Itching after hot baths. Skin of the face and extremities becomes bluish-red. Some redness of the mucous membranes, particularly of the eye. Of unknown cause. Stems from an overgrowth of blood-forming tissues in the bone marrow, resulting in excessive amounts of red cells in the blood, with a thickening of the blood and an increased tendency to clotting.

WHAT TO DO

- **Consult your physician immediately.** If long untreated, can lead to stroke and gastrointestinal hemorrhages.
- For treatment, phlebotomy (bloodletting) may be used to reduce blood thickness and the number of red cells. Medication may be prescribed to control the overproduction of red cells.

PURPURA, IDIOPATHIC THROMBOCYTOPENIC

SYMPTOMS

Small, round, purplish-red spots formed by bleeding into the skin, which turn into black-and-blue marks. Nosebleeds. Bleeding in the gastrointestinal or urinary tract. A disease of unknown cause in which platelets, small bodies in the blood that help prevent bleeding, are removed too rapidly by the spleen. A kind of purpura much like and with the same symptoms as idiopathic thrombocytopenic may result from a drug such as quinine, quinidine or chlorothiazide. It will disappear when drug use is stopped. The purpura may also stem from an infection such as measles or infectious mononucleosis and will disappear when the infection does.

WHAT TO DO

- **Consult your physician.**
- Occasionally the disorder disappears on its own. In some cases, medication may be prescribed to reduce bleeding and increase the number of platelets. If the disorder persists and is severe, surgery may be recommended.

SICKLE-CELL ANEMIA

SYMPTOMS

May include any or many of the symptoms for iron deficiency anemia (see ANEMIA FROM IRON DEFICIENCY), but are usually more severe. Often include: Jaundice (skin yellowing). Episodes of joint pain. Intermittent fever. Intermittent severe abdominal pain with vomiting. Episodes of back pain. An inherited form of hemolytic anemia, mainly affecting blacks. Red blood cells are distorted, becoming sickle-shaped instead of round, and are fragile and easily destroyed.

WHAT TO DO

- **Consult your physician.**
- No specific medication is available as yet, but leads are being followed in increasingly intensive research. Meanwhile, treatment is for symptoms. Transfusion may be recommended to interrupt a cycle of closely spaced acute episodes.

BRAIN, SPINE & NERVOUS SYSTEM

BELL'S PALSY

SYMPTOMS

May begin with: Pain behind the ear. Followed within hours by: Facial weakness on one side. Some facial paralysis. Inability to smile. Inability to close the eye on the affected side. Difficulty speaking and eating. The disease is a neuritis, an inflammation of the facial nerve that controls expression. The cause is unknown but may involve injury to or pressure on the nerve.

WHAT TO DO

- **Consult your physician.** Complete recovery within several months is likely, especially with medical help.
- To protect an exposed eye, medicated drops or patching may be prescribed. Electrical stimulation and physical therapy may be recommended.

BRAIN TUMORS

SYMPTOMS

Highly variable because there are many types of tumors which may occur in various areas of the brain. May begin with: Mild but slowly progressive

disturbances in sight, smell or balance. Weakness in leg or arm muscles. Further symptoms may include: **Headache. Vomiting. Personality changes. Convulsive seizures. Drowsiness. Lethargy. Disordered conduct. Mental impairment.** Of unknown cause. May occur at any age, but most common in early adult or middle life.

WHAT TO DO

• **Consult your physician immediately at any slight suspicion of brain tumor.** Headaches, of course, are common, but seek medical help if they develop suddenly and there is no history of chronic headaches.

• Brain tumors are not invariably hopeless. More than a third are benign — not cancerous. Even many malignant tumors can be treated with success.

• Surgical removal is increasingly possible because of advances in surgical techniques.

ENCEPHALITIS (Sleeping sickness)

SYMPTOMS

Fever (to 106°F./40.1°C. in infants; to 103°F./39.4°C. in older children and adults). Severe headache. Drowsiness, possibly extending to stupor. Vomiting. Stiff neck. Sometimes: Muscle twitching. Confusion. Convulsions. Coma. Paralysis of the extremities. An acute brain inflammation caused by viruses. Occasionally may develop as a complication of measles, flu, chicken pox or whopping cough.

WHAT TO DO

• **Consult your physician.**

• No specific drugs for the disease are available. Supportive measures directed by the physician may include bed rest, cold compresses and intravenous feeding. Complete recovery is usual.

EPILEPSY

SYMPTOMS

Brief or prolonged loss of consciousness. Involuntary movements. GRAND MAL type of seizure may be heralded by a warning: Ringing in the ears. Spots before the eyes. Tingling in the fingers. Followed by: An outcry. Loss of consciousness. Falling. Muscle contractions. Loss of bladder control. Loss of bowel control. An attack usually lasts 2 to 5 minutes. May be followed by: Sleep. Headache. Muscle soreness. PETIT MAL, occurring predominantly in children, is manifested by: Loss of consciousness for 10 to 30 seconds. No falling. Twitching about the eyes and mouth. Temporary cessation of activity. PSYCHOMOTOR (temporal lobe) seizures produce: Clouding of consciousness for 1 or 2 minutes. Repeated purposeless movements (such as hand-clapping). Staring. Staggering. Mental confusion.

Epilepsy is a disorder of brain function, affecting almost 2 million Americans, who are otherwise normal. Mental deterioration is rare.

WHAT TO DO

• **Consult your physician.**

• Many anticonvulsant drugs are available for treatment. They allow significant or even total control for the majority of patients, enabling them to live virtually normal lives.

HEADACHES: CLUSTER

SYMPTOMS

Excruciating burning and boring pain, involving the regions of the eye, temple, neck, and often the face. Eye tearing. Runny nose. Nose obstruction. Sweating. Cluster headaches last less than an hour. They appear suddenly, occurring as often as several times a day for weeks or months, then disappear suddenly, and may reappear months or years later. They are 5 times more common in men than women.

WHAT TO DO

• **Consult your physician.**

• Treatment may include some drugs used for migraine or other kinds of headaches.

• Recent reports indicate oxygen administered by face mask often relieves a cluster headache in 5 to 10 minutes.

HEADACHES: MIGRAINE

SYMPTOMS

In one form (CLASSICAL MIGRAINE): Flashing lights and other visual disturbances occur half an hour or more before the headache. Pain, often on one side of the head, is aching or throbbing, beating with the pulse. Often accompanied by: Nausea. Vomiting. In another form (COMMON MIGRAINE): No advance visual phenomena. Pain is more often on both sides of the head rather than just on one side. Migraine is much more common in women than in men. Heredity may be involved; about 75 percent of migraine patients have family histories of the headaches.

WHAT TO DO

• **Consult your physician.**

• Medication, including newer drugs, may be prescribed to help prevent or reduce the frequency of attacks. Often, it helps to avoid some foods which act on blood vessels, a major factor in migraine. These foods include: aged or strong cheese (particularly cheddar), pickled herring, chicken livers, pods of broad beans, canned figs, alcohol and in some cases cured meats containing nitrites (frankfurters, bacon, ham, salami).

• Helpful and increasingly in use: biofeedback techniques, which teach how to avert attacks through the temporary use of electronic sensing equipment.

• Consulting a nutritionist can be helpful.

HEADACHES: TENSION

SYMPTOMS

Dull, persistent head pain. May last for several hours. May occur daily or several times a week or month. Can feel like a tight hatband around the head. The most common kind of headache. Related to chronic muscular contraction about the head and neck. May be brought on either by biologic stress (uncomfortable body position, eyestrain, arthritis of the neck area) or emotional stress (anxiety, frustration, boredom, depression).

WHAT TO DO

• For an occasional tension headache, moist heat and massage may be helpful.
• **For chronic tension headache, consult your physician.** Continued use of a pain-reliever may lead to rebound headaches from the medication. If depression contributes to the headache, antidepressant medication may be prescribed.
• Helpful and increasingly in use: biofeedback techniques, which teach how to relax contracting muscles through the temporary use of electronic sensing equipment.

HEADACHES: OTHER

In women, variants of tension or migraine headaches may occur before and during menstruation, during menopause and immediately after sexual intercourse. They may be related to hormonal events in the body, anxiety or exertion. Consultation with a physician can provide reassurance.

Oral contraceptives may also produce headaches in some women. Your physician may prescribe another type of oral contraceptive or another means of birth control.

Men and women who consume a lot of caffeine at work during the week (in coffee, tea, cola drinks, etc.) may experience headaches over the weekend when they reduce their consumption and undergo caffeine withdrawal.

MENINGITIS

SYMPTOMS

May begin with: A cold or other respiratory illness or a sore throat. Followed within 24 hours or less by: Fever. Headache. Stiff neck. Vomiting. Irritability. Confusion. Drowsiness. Stupor. Coma. An inflammation of the membranes (meninges) covering the brain and spinal cord caused by infection by bacteria, viruses or fungi. An epidemic type, **MENINGOCOCCEMIA,** caused by meningococcal bacteria, is highly contagious because the organisms are present in the throat as well as in the cerebrospinal fluid. **TUBERCULOUS MENINGITIS** is produced by the same organisms that cause lung TB. **ASEPTIC MENINGITIS,** mainly a disease of young children during the summer months, is caused by viruses, most commonly mumps and polio.

WHAT TO DO

• **Consult your physician immediately.** Meningitis is a serious disease, once 90 percent fatal, now almost always responsive to prompt treatment.
• A spinal tap — for study of organisms in the spinal fluid — helps diagnosis and can pinpoint the causative kind of organism.
• Antibiotics may be prescribed. Supportive therapy may include administration of fluids and other medication.

MULTIPLE SCLEROSIS

SYMPTOMS

May begin with mild early symptoms such as: Slight vision disturbances. Fatigue in the arms or legs. Some difficulty with urination or bladder control. Mild emotional upsets. Later symptoms may include one or more of the following: Double vision. Loss of part of the visual field. Weakness. Fatigue. Tremors. Impaired balance. Unsteady walking. Gait stiffness. Slowed speech. Increased difficulties with bladder control. Difficulties with bowel control. Paralysis may develop in any part of the body. The cause of MS is unknown, but it usually affects young adults. Involves development of hardened patches in the brain and spinal cord, affecting nerve activity.

WHAT TO DO

• **Consult your physician.** MS has a variable course, with ups and downs, improvements and worsenings. No specific treatment is available, but muscle wastage and invalidism can be postponed, often even prevented.
• Physical therapy, muscle training, exercise and massage are helpful.

NEURALGIA, TRIGEMINAL
(Tic douloureux)

SYMPTOMS

Episodes of intense facial pain, stabbing or lightning-like, along the trigeminal (fifth cranial) nerve, leading from the brain to the face and jaw. The pain may extend from the forehead to the lips, nose, tongue and gums. Often set off by chewing,

brushing teeth or talking. **Episodes are brief, lasting a minute or two. They first occur at intervals of weeks or months, then later with increasing frequency.** The cause is unknown; there is no evidence of organic change in the nerve. Most often affects older people.

WHAT TO DO
- **Consult your physician.** Heat or cold may provide some relief. Medication and other medical measures may be prescribed.

PARKINSON'S DISEASE

SYMPTOMS

Often begin with: A tremor in a hand. Followed by: Increasing tremors which may involve much or all of the body. Fixed facial expression. Unblinking eyes. Drooling. Stiffened muscles. Shuffling gait. Other symptoms may include: Cramplike pains in the limbs and spine. Depression. Mild dementia. A chronic central nervous system disorder of unknown cause that occurs in the middle-aged and elderly. Similar symptoms may result from certain drugs (such as strong tranquilizers) used for extensive periods, poisoning by carbon monoxide or manganese, and brain injury.

WHAT TO DO
- **Consult your physician.** Although there is no cure, medical treatment is effective for relief.

SCIATICA

SYMPTOMS

Severe pain that may begin in the buttock and ex- tend down the back of the thigh and lower leg to the ankle. An inflammation of the sciatic nerve, one of the longest in the body, extending from the base of the spine down the thigh to the lower leg and foot. May be caused by osteoarthritis of the lower spine or rupture of a spinal disk, causing pressure on the root of the nerve in the spine. Occasionally may be induced by diabetes or a vitamin deficiency.

WHAT TO DO
- **Consult your physician.**
- **Conservative treatment often helps.** May include use of a firm mattress and local heat. Medication may be prescribed. Traction may be helpful. When necessary, surgery may be recommended to remove the ruptured disk.

TICS (Habit spasms)

SYMPTOMS

Sudden, brief, repetitive, purposeless movements such as twitching of the corner of the eye or mouth, head nodding or shaking, throat clearing, shoulder shrugging. Tics typically begin about age 6 and tend to disappear around puberty, but they may persist into adulthood. Sometimes associated with encephalitis. Mostly of unknown cause though often attributed to psychological mechanisms.
NOTE: Gilles de la Tourette's syndrome, starting in childhood with blinking, grimaces, shoulder shrugging, arm movements, may progress in teenage years to grunting, sniffing, shouting, barking noises and compulsive swearing. Of unknown cause, it does not affect the intelligence.

WHAT TO DO
- **Consult your physician.**

CANCER

BLADDER CANCER

SYMPTOMS

Often begin with: Frequent urination accompanied by burning or pain. Blood and pus in the urine. Later: A mass in the abdomen may be felt on examination. Affects men twice as often as women. Known causes include aniline dyes and, possibly, tobacco tar products excreted in the urine.

WHAT TO DO
- **Consult your physician immediately.** Many cases of bladder cancer can be treated effectively, the earlier the better.

BONE CANCER

SYMPTOMS

Persistent or progressive pain in a bone, later followed by swelling. Cancer can spread to a bone from other sites, most often from the lung, breast, prostate, kidney and thyroid. Or it may arise originally in the bone, especially in children and young adults. Most common sites: the knee, thigh, upper arm, pelvis, ribs. The cause is unknown.

WHAT TO DO
- **Consult your physician promptly for persistent bone pain.**

BRAIN CANCER

SYMPTOMS

Any or many of the following, depending upon the location of the growth: **Headache. Nausea. Vomiting. Convulsive seizures. Drowsiness. Lethargy. Personality changes. Mental impairment. Muscle weakness. Failing vision. Loss of balance and coordination. Tremors. Paralysis. Hearing impairment in one ear. Ringing in the ears.** May occur at any age but most common in early adult or middle life. The cause is unknown.

WHAT TO DO

• **Consult your physician promptly for any symptoms that could indicate brain cancer.** They may or may not do so. Early diagnosis and treatment are vital.

BREAST CANCER

SYMPTOMS

Slowly growing, painless mass or lump in the breast. Other symptoms may include: Elevated or retracted nipple. Distortion of breast contour. Dimpling of skin over the growth. Pitting of breast skin producing an orange-skin appearance. The most common malignancy in women, it occurs in only a very small percentage of men. Rare before age 30; climbing incidence after menopause.

WHAT TO DO

• **Consult your physician immediately.** Most breast lumps are found by women themselves. Most are not cancerous. But early diagnosis can be vital for increasing chances of cure.

CERVICAL CANCER

SYMPTOMS

Often begin with: **Slight vaginal discharge that is watery or contains blood. May occur especially after intercourse. Other early symptoms may include: Vaginal bleeding. Spotting. Irregular menstruation. Later symptoms may include: Constipation. Vomiting. Lower back pain. Weight loss. Urinary disturbances.** The third most frequent malignancy among women, after breast and skin cancers. High incidence among women with histories of early and frequent intercourse and multiple sexual partners.

WHAT TO DO

• **Consult your physician immediately.** Diagnosed and treated early, cervical cancer has a high rate of cure.
• The Pap smear test can detect 95 percent of early cervical cancers. It has more than halved the number of deaths and could eliminate most fatalities if used by all women. (Fewer than 40 percent now have an annual test.)

COLON AND RECTAL CANCER

SYMPTOMS

Any or all of the following: **Bloody stool. Change in the bowel habits from few movements to many or many to few. Narrowing of stools. Cramps. Other symptoms may include: Anemia. Weight loss. Weakness.** Among the most common malignancies, cancers of the colon and rectum mostly occur in middle life and later years. The cause is unknown, although there is some suggestion that it may involve excessive meat intake and inadequate fiber or bulk in the diet.

WHAT TO DO

• **Consult your physician immediately at any indication of possible colon or rectal cancer.** Cure rates of 80 to 90 percent are possible with early detection and treatment.

ESOPHAGUS CANCER

SYMPTOMS

May begin with: **A sensation of food (especially of soft bread or meat) sticking behind the breastbone. Boring pain may occur with swallowing or be persistent. Weight loss develops.** About 1 percent of all cancers occur in the esophagus, mostly after age 50. The cause is unknown. Under suspicion: smoking, excessive use of alcohol, hot and spicy foods.

WHAT TO DO

• **Consult your physician immediately at any possible indication of cancer of the esophagus.** Early symptoms are often ignored. The cancer is extremely dangerous.

GALLBLADDER CANCER

SYMPTOMS

Similar to those of gallstones: **Upper abdominal discomfort. Bloating. Belching. Nausea (especially after eating fatty foods). Jaundice (skin yellowing). Weakness.** Gallbladder cancer is relatively rare and occurs mostly in older people. It is usually discovered during the course of surgery for gallstones.

WHAT TO DO

• **Consult your physician.**

HODGKIN'S DISEASE

SYMPTOMS

May begin with: **Intense itching. Another early symptom: Painless enlargement of the lymph nodes, often first on one side of the neck and then the other, then later on under the arms and in the groin.** As the disease progresses, later symptoms may include: **Sweating. Fever. Weakness. Appetite loss. Weight loss. Bone pain. Swelling in the legs or elsewhere.** The cancerous disease is rare in children under 10 and occurs with equal frequency among young and older adults. It is about 1.4 times more frequent among men than women. The cause is unknown; an infectious organism is suspected but not proved.

WHAT TO DO
- Consult your physician.

KIDNEY CANCER

SYMPTOMS

Often begin with: Blood in the urine. Other symptoms include: Flank pain. An abdominal mass. Fever. Kidney cancer makes up 1 to 2 percent of adult cancers. It also occurs in children; see **KIDNEY CANCER (Wilms' tumor).** About two-thirds of the adults affected are men. The cause is unknown.

WHAT TO DO
- Consult your physician.

KIDNEY CANCER (Wilms' tumor)

SYMPTOMS

Often begin with: An abdominal mass discovered in the child by a parent or physician. Followed by: Pain. Fever. Appetite loss. Nausea. Vomiting. Blood in the urine. The tumor actually begins before birth, lies dormant, then usually manifests itself before the fifth year. The cause is unknown.

WHAT TO DO
- Consult your physician.
- Response to treatment is often excellent. Cure rates have gone beyond 50 percent, reaching up to 90 percent in some reports.

LARYNX CANCER

SYMPTOMS

An early major symptom: Persistent, painless hoarseness. Further symptoms may include: Swallowing difficulty. Breathing difficulty. Coughing. Cancer of the larynx occurs mostly in men, usually over 50 years old. Appears to be related to smoking and consumption of alcohol.

WHAT TO DO
- Consult your physician.
- Early cases often can be treated effectively.

LEUKEMIA

SYMPTOMS

Symptoms of ACUTE LEUKEMIA may include: Abrupt high fever. Infection of the mouth, throat or lungs. Joint pains. Purplish-red skin bruises and sores. Bleeding from the mouth or nose. Bloody stool. Blood in the urine. In some cases, the disease begins insidiously with increasing pallor and weakness. **Symptoms of CHRONIC LEUKEMIA may include: Increasing weakness. Fatigue. Appetite loss. Swollen lymph nodes. Pallor. Weight loss. Vague upper abdominal distress or heaviness. Breastbone tenderness.** The leukemias are malignant disorders of the blood-forming tissues leading to abnormally high production of white blood cells and the crowding out of other important blood elements. Some leukemias in chickens, mice and rats are due to viruses; there is no proof of such origin in humans. Although the acute and chronic forms may occur at any age, the acute primarily affects children and the chronic primarily affects adults over 30.

WHAT TO DO
- Consult your physician.

LIP CANCER

SYMPTOMS

A blister or sore, usually on the lower lip, that fails to heal and tends to bleed easily. More common in older people, more in men than women. May result from exposure to the sun, or from pipe and cigar smoking.

WHAT TO DO
- Consult your physician.

LIVER CANCER

SYMPTOMS

Abdominal pain. A mass in the right upper quarter of the abdomen. Weight loss. A possible later symptom: Jaundice (skin yellowing). Cancer originating in the liver is rare in the U.S. but common in Africa and the Orient. At least half the cases in the U.S. are associated with cirrhosis of the liver. Cancer originating elsewhere in the body — in the gastrointestinal tract, pancreas, gallbladder, lung or breast — may spread to the liver.

WHAT TO DO
- Consult your physician.

LUNG CANCER

SYMPTOMS

**May begin with: A new cough or a change in the

severity or character of a chronic cough. Followed by: Coughing up of blood or bloody sputum. Wheezing or other chest noises. Chest ache or pain. Shortness of breath. In later stages: Appetite loss. Weight loss. Weakness. Hoarseness. The most common cancer in men, but increasing in women. Occurs mostly after age 40. Smoking is a major factor. Pollution may also be involved.

WHAT TO DO
- **Consult your physician immediately.** Unfortunately, most cases are inoperable when diagnosed, often because of delay.

MALIGNANT MELANOMA

SYMPTOMS

A pigmented mole or other pigmented area of the skin or mucous membrane suddenly increases size, darkens, ulcerates and bleeds. Although very rare, especially in children, melanomas are a little more frequent in pregnant than nonpregnant women. Some can be exceedingly dangerous because they spread rapidly. The cause is unknown.

WHAT TO DO
- **Consult your physician.**

MOUTH CANCER

SYMPTOMS

To be safe, any sore on the tongue, gum, palate, cheek, floor of the mouth or other site that fails to heal in 2 weeks, or any white patch that replaces the normal pink color of the tongue or inside of the mouth should be regarded as cancerous until proved otherwise by microscopic examination of a small sample (biopsy). Possible at any age, mouth cancer more often affects older people, men more than women. Smoking and high alcohol intake are suspected factors.

WHAT TO DO
- **Consult your physician immediately.**
- Early treatment is effective.

MULTIPLE MYELOMA
(Bone marrow cancer)

SYMPTOMS

Persistent, unexplained bone pain, especially in the back or chest. Repeated bacterial infections, especially pneumonia. Weakness. Fatigue. Bone fractures. Usually affects people over 40, men twice as often as women. Commonly fatal.

WHAT TO DO
- **Consult your physician.**

NEUROBLASTOMA
(Nervous system malignancy)

SYMPTOMS

An abdominal mass that is firm but not tender. Further symptoms may include: Breathing difficulty. Obstruction of the urine flow. Weight loss. Fever. Anemia. Lymph node enlargement. The most common solid tumor of childhood. Arises from the nervous system or nerve cells of the adrenal gland. The cause is unknown.

WHAT TO DO
- **Consult your physician.**

NON-HODGKIN'S LYMPHOMA

SYMPTOMS

Lymph nodes become rubbery. Tonsils may be involved. Other symptoms depend upon the organs affected: Sometimes they resemble the symptoms of cancer of the stomach or small intestine; see STOMACH CANCER and SMALL INTESTINE CANCER. Later symptoms: Weight loss. Fever. Night sweats. Weakness. In some cases, a disease resembling leukemia develops; see LEUKEMIA. More frequent than Hodgkin's disease, Non-Hodgkin's Lymphoma can occur at any age. The cause is unknown; a viral origin is suspected.

WHAT TO DO
- **Consult your physician.**

OVARIAN CANCER

SYMPTOMS

Begin with: Vague lower abdominal discomfort. Mild digestive upsets. Possible abnormal vaginal bleeding. Later symptoms may include: Abdominal swelling. Pelvic pain. Anemia. Emaciation. Peak incidence is in the 50's. The cause is unknown.

WHAT TO DO
- **Consult your physician.**
- Treatment depends upon the size of the tumor and whether it extends beyond the ovary.

PANCREAS CANCER

SYMPTOMS

A major symptom: Abdominal pain that often

spreads to the back, and is relieved by sitting up or bending forward. **Other symptoms: Jaundice (skin yellowing). Appetite loss. Weight loss. Nausea. Vomiting (sometimes with bloody vomit). Constipation. Diarrhea. Stools sometimes darkened by blood pigments.** Most often occurs late in life. The cause is unknown.

WHAT TO DO

• **Consult your physician.**

PHARYNX (THROAT) CANCER

SYMPTOMS

Depend upon the location of the cancer. Symptoms of a nasal obstruction or obstruction of the eustachian tube leading to the ear: Ear disturbances. Bloody nasal discharge. Possible symptom of an affected tonsil. A sore throat with pain spreading to the ear on the affected side. Other symptoms may include: Breathing difficulty. Swallowing difficulty. Nasal speech. Bad breath. Facial paralysis. Sever pain in the throat. A mass in the neck.

WHAT TO DO

• **Consult your physician immediately.** Too often, cancer of the pharynx is not diagnosed until it has spread.

PROSTATE CANCER

SYMPTOMS

Increasing difficulty urinating. Increasingly frequent urination. Diminished stream. Sometimes: Blood in the urine. Later: Bone pain. Symptoms are similar to those of nonmalignant enlargement of the prostate but call for medical diagnosis. Prostate cancer accounts for the majority of malignancies in men over 65, but may occur at younger ages.

WHAT TO DO

• **Consult your physician.**
• Early, still localized cases can often be cured.

RETINA CANCER (Retinoblastoma)

SYMPTOMS

May begin with: Whitishness of the pupil of the eye. Squinting. A congenital tumor, often diagnosed before age 2. Responsible for 2 percent of all childhood malignancies. Affects both eyes in about 25 percent of the cases.

WHAT TO DO

• **Consult your physician.**
• Most early cases can be cured.

SKIN CANCER

SYMPTOMS

Depend upon the type of cancer. BASAL CELL CARCINOMA, non-spreading, begins as a small, pale papule or solid elevation, usually on an exposed skin site, then slowly enlarges and shows a central ulcer. SQUAMOUS CELL CARCINOMA, which tends to spread, appears as a small reddish papule or patch, then after months or years begins to grow, forming a crusted ulcer with hard edges. It may then spread rapidly to the mouth, nose or vulva as well as on the skin. (Also see **MALIGNANT MELANOMA**). The most common and readily curable malignancy, skin cancer seems to be related to excessive exposure to sunlight, x-ray, coal tar, nickel, beryllium and arsenic. Light-skinned people are most susceptible.

WHAT TO DO

• **Consult your physician.** To be safe, inquire about any sore or ulcer that fails to heal promptly, or a mole that suddenly changes color, size or texture.

SMALL INTESTINE CANCER

SYMPTOMS

Intermittent, crampy midabdominal pain. Stools darkened by blood pigment. Anemia. A rare tumor, unlike cancer of the colon or large intestine. The cause is unknown.

WHAT TO DO

• **Consult your physician.**

STOMACH CANCER

SYMPTOMS

Upper abdominal discomfort, sometimes worsening after even small meals. Vague pain over the pit of the stomach. Appetite loss. Weight loss. Vomiting. Anemia. The symptoms may occur singly or in combination. Stomach cancer has been decreasing and is relatively rare in the U.S., though it is still common in Japan and some other countries. It tends to occur in the later years, more often in men than women. The cause is unknown, though contributing factors may include aflotoxin, (a cancer-producing agent in contaminated food), smoked fish, alcohol and deficiencies in vitamin A and magnesium. Pernicious anemia may predispose to stomach cancer.

- **Consult your physician immediately.** Early diagnosis is vital.

TESTIS CANCER

SYMPTOMS

A mass can be felt in the scrotum. Over time, it increases in size. It may or may not be painful. Most commonly affects young men 20 to 30, but may occur at other ages. Testicular self-examination can be a key factor in early detection. It should be as widely practiced among men as breast examination is among women.

WHAT TO DO

- **Consult your physician immediately.** Especially when detected early, testicular cancer is one of the most curable malignancies.

THYROID CANCER

SYMPTOMS

A mass in the neck, usually without pain or tenderness. When soft, mobile and made up of many nodules, the tumor may be benign. When hard, irregular and fixed, it may be malignant. Tests are necessary to make the differentiation. Thyroid cancer is more common in women than men.

WHAT TO DO

- **Consult your physician.**

UTERINE CANCER

SYMPTOMS

Vaginal bleeding. Odorous discharge. Possible menstrual irregularities (often several heavy flows followed by none, then the return of menses). Later symptoms may include: Constipation. Lower back or abdominal pain. Urinary irregularities. Cancer of the uterus is most common between ages 50 and 60. Predisposing factors may include delayed menopause, disturbed menstrual history, infertility, obesity, high blood pressure, diabetes and a family history of breast or ovarian cancer.

WHAT TO DO

- **Consult your physician.**

VAGINAL CANCER

SYMPTOMS

Bleeding after intercourse. In some cases, vaginal bleeding at other times. If the bladder or rectum become involved, other symptoms may include: Painful intercourse. Watery discharge. Frequent and urgent urination. Painful defecation. Vaginal cancer is most common from age 45 to 65.

WHAT TO DO

- **Consult your physician.**

CHILDHOOD DISORDERS

CEREBRAL PALSY

SYMPTOMS

Vary. The gradations range from minor awkwardness of gait or slight speech impairment to: Distortion of the body. Inability to learn readily. Visual defects. Seizures. Inability to walk. Inability to talk. In severly afflicted children, certain symptoms may be present from birth: Vomiting. Irritability. Nursing difficulty. In milder cases,these symptoms may not be apparent until the second or third year when the child fails to develop normal motor skills such as sitting up, crawling and walking. Up to 0.1 percent of all children and up to 1 percent of premature babies have cerebral palsy. The disability involves damage to the central nervous system that may result from disorders in the womb, birth injury or lack of sufficient oxygen at or about birth. There are three major forms, depending upon the brain areas affected: **SPASTIC,** with stiffness and movement difficulty. **ATHETOID,** with uncontrollable, purposeless movements and writhings. **ATACTIC,** with poor coordination and balance, and a staggering gait.

WHAT TO DO

- **Consult your physician.**
- The goal of the treatment is maximum independence within the individual child's capabilities. Treatment necessarily varies depending upon individual needs but may include any or many of the following: medication, orthopedic surgery, casts, braces, special exercises, muscle training, speech training.

CHICKEN POX (Varicella)

SYMPTOMS

During the third week after exposure may begin with: Mild headache. Moderate fever. Malaise. A day or two later, small red spots develop, usually first on the back and chest. These spots enlarge after several hours, each forming a blister in the center filled with clear fluid. After another day or two, the fluid turns yellow. Crusts or scabs then form, which peel off in 5 to 20 days. During this time there may be severe itching. Caused by the same virus that produces shingles. Incubation: 2 weeks or a little more. Period of contagion: about 2 weeks. No vaccine is available.

WHAT TO DO
- **Consult your physician.**
- Most cases are mild and need treatment only to relieve symptoms. Wet compresses help control itching.
- To avoid complicating infections from scratching: Keep the child's hands clean and nails clipped. Bathe him frequently in soap and water.

CLEFT LIP/PALATE

SYMPTOMS

Obvious malformation. The defect may be limited to the outer flesh of the upper lip extending to the nostril — a "harelip," so-called because it suggests the lip of a rabbit — or may extend back through the midline of the upper jaw and through the roof of the mouth. Sometimes only the soft palate, located at the rear of the mouth, is involved. An afflicted infant may have difficulty nursing because the opening between his mouth and nose prevents suction. Cleft lips or palates, which occur in about 1 of every 700 births, result from the failure of the two sides of the face to unite properly at an early stage of prenatal development.

WHAT TO DO
- **Consult your physician.**
- Immediate feeding can be accomplished with a dropper, cup or spoon — or an obdurator may be used. This is an appliance which closes the cleft while the baby is nursing.
- Surgery to close a cleft lip can usually be carried out not long after birth. A cleft palate can usually be reconstructed before the child learns to talk — at a year to 18 months. Often the plastic surgeon works in consultation with a dentist, orthodontist, speech specialist and other experts. In most cases, the properly treated child will have a normal appearance, speech and manner.

COLIC

SYMPTOMS

Paroxysms of crying. Irritability. Apparent abdominal pain. The legs are drawn up and bent to the abdomen. Abdominal distension. May begin shortly after the infant is brought home from the hospital and persist for 3 to 4 months. Not a disease in itself, colic can be symptomatic of any of a wide range of problems: Swallowed air, under- or over-feeding, intolerance of some foods, intestinal disorder.

WHAT TO DO
- **Consult your physician.**
- **After ruling out any underlying problems, the physician may suggest improved burping technique, smaller and more frequent feedings, a change in formula, rocking.**

CYSTIC FIBROSIS

SYMPTOMS

May begin with: Delay in regaining birth weight despite a good appetite. Other early symptoms may include: Chronic cough. Rapid breathing. Large and foul-smelling stools. Protruberant abdomen. Respiratory infections. Coughing and vomiting paroxysms. Barrel-like chest. Bluish color. An inherited disease affecting the pancreas, sweat glands and respiratory system. Cystic fibrosis occurs in about 1 in 1500 births. The cause is unknown. It is also called pancreatic cystic fibrosis, fibrocystic disease of the pancreas and mucoviscidosis.

WHAT TO DO
- **Consult your physician.**
- No cure is available, but treatment can often improve the health and extend life. It may include replacement of pancreatic enzymes, careful diet, mist tents to help liquefy mucus during sleep, breathing exercises, postural drainage, medication.

DIPHTHERIA

SYMPTOMS

Begin with: A mild sore throat. Progress to: Fever of 100° to 104°F./37.7° to 40°C. Headache. Nausea. Swallowing difficulty. Prostration may follow. A grayish membrane may appear in the throat or nose, causing breathing and swallowing difficulty. Incubation period is 1 to 4 days. Spread by coughing and sneezing and by handkerchiefs, towels, utensils and other objects used by an infected person.

WHAT TO DO
- **Consult your physician.**
- Treated by injection of an antitoxin that will counteract the toxic reaction from the causative bacteria. Bed rest is necessary, along with careful nursing and staying alert for possible airway obstruction. Antibiotics are often used.
- Diphtheria can be prevented by vaccination with DPT (diphtheria, pertussis, tetanus). The vaccine should be given to all infants.

GERMAN MEASLES (Rubella)

SYMPTOMS

Begin with: Malaise. Lymph node swelling behind the ears and in back of the neck. Fever. Slight cold and sore throat. Progress to: A light rose-colored rash on the face and neck that quickly spreads to the trunk and extremities. A flush may also appear, particularly on the face. The rash usually lasts about 3 days. A mild viral disease, German measles can have serious effects if contracted by a woman during the early months of pregnancy. In that circumstance, it may cause stillbirth, abortion or congenital defects in the child.

WHAT TO DO

• **Consult your physician.**
• Treatment is usually not needed.
• German measles can be prevented by vaccination. The vaccine should be given to all children, especially to girls long before they reach childbearing age.

MEASLES (Rubeola)

SYMPTOMS

Begin with: Fever. Runny nose. Hacking cough. Reddened eyes. 2 to 4 days later, Koplik's spots—resembling grains of sand surrounded by rosy areas—appear on the inner surface of the cheeks opposite the 1st and 2nd upper molars. A sore throat also develops. 3 to 5 days after the start of symptoms, the characteristic rash appears. It begins in front of and below the ears and on the side of the neck, then spreads downward and covers the entire body in about 36 hours. At first, the rash consists of separate pink spots about one-quarter inch in diameter. Later, the spots may run together. In 3 to 5 days, the fever (which at peak may reach 104°F./40°C. or higher) falls and the rash begins to fade rapidly. Incubation period is 7 to 14 days. Highly contagious. Spread by droplets from the nose, throat or mouth. Although measles is usually benign, there can be dangerous complications: pneumonia, middle ear and other infections, encephalitis.

WHAT TO DO

• **Consult your physician.**
• Treatment may consist of fluids, medication and confinement to bed during the fever to prevent complications.
• Itching may be relieved with calamine lotion.
• After exposure, an unvaccinated child or adult who has not had measles may be protected by gamma globulin injection or by vaccine given within 2 days of exposure.
• Measles can be prevented by vaccination.

MENTAL RETARDATION

SYMPTOMS

During infancy, symptoms which may suggest possible subaverage intellectual ability include: **Marked lethargy. Marked lack of responsiveness to the environment. Marked slowness at feeding skills, head-lifting, reaching for objects, sitting.** The birthrate for children with IQs under 50 is 36 per 10,000 live births. In 80 percent of the cases, the cause is unknown. The remainder are attributable to many possible causes, including chromosomal abnormalities, hereditary disorders and viral infections in the womb. Complications at or about birth — such as bleeding, breech or high forceps delivery, breathing difficulty — may increase the risk. Premature babies weighing less than 3.3 pounds have some increased risk.

WHAT TO DO

• **Consult your physician.**
• Accurate diagnosis requires thorough physical examination, evaluation of the child's development and brain wave and other tests. Developmental delays — in sitting, walking, drawing, writing, etc. — may also be due to neuromuscular disorders or emotional problems.
• Treatment may include correction of any contributory problems such as thyroid deficiency, development of a program for education, psychological support.

MINIMAL BRAIN DYSFUNCTION (Learning disorders)

SYMPTOMS

Before school age, parents may notice: Hyperactivity. Impulsiveness. Emotional instability. Lack of motor coordination. Later symptoms: Discipline problems. Short attention span. Easily distracted. General inability to control impulses. Constant moving, touching and handling. May have perceptual problems such as difficulty judging distance, reversal of numerals and letters. Failure in schoolwork or uneven achievement. It is estimated that 5 to 15 percent of American schoolchildren (2.5 to 7.5 million) have some type of learning disorder. There is no single cause. Because 5 times as many boys as girls have learning disorders, some may be genetically sex-linked. In some cases, nervous system disorders are present; in others, there are emotional problems.

WHAT TO DO

• **Consult your physician.** A multidisciplinary team approach to diagnosis may be needed, with the physician participating along with a neurologist, psychologist, parents and teachers.
• Treatment includes management of any specific medical problems and help with educational difficulties. In some cases, remedial school work may be needed.

MUMPS

SYMPTOMS

Begin with: Chilly sensations. Headache. Appetite

loss. **Malaise. Low to moderate fever. Followed in 12 to 24 hours by: Swelling of one, or more commonly, both the salivary glands under the jaw or in front of or below the ear. Pain on chewing or swallowing. Temperature often rises to 103° or 104°F./39.4° or 40°C. After about a week: Gland swelling may disappear. In boys past puberty: Testes may become inflamed.** A viral disease, less communicable than measles and chicken pox. Most often affects children 5 to 15.

WHAT TO DO
- **Consult your physician.**
- Treatment may include bed rest (especially for children after puberty), soft diet, medication. If the testes are involved, to help avoid tension, the scrotum may be supported in cotton on an adhesive tape bridge between the thighs. Ice packs may help relieve pain.
- One attack confers immunity. A preventive vaccine is available.

MUSCULAR DYSTROPHY

SYMPTOMS

In the most common type (DUCHENNE) typically affecting boys 3 to 7, muscular weakness causes: Waddling gait. Toe-walking. Frequent falls. Difficulty standing and climbing stairs. Calves increase in size. By age 10 or 12, most patients are confined to wheelchairs. In another, less common type (FACIOSCAPULOHUMERAL): The muscles of the face and shoulder girdle are predominantly affected, beginning in adolescence. The face becomes expressionless. The arms cannot be lifted above the head. Of unknown cause, muscular dystrophies are hereditary and progressive. For the facioscapulohumeral form, life expectancy is normal.

WHAT TO DO
- **Consult your physician.**
- No specific treatment. But exercise — if necessary, passive exercise — can extend ambulation in more severe cases. Corrective surgery may sometimes be recommended.

POLIOMYELITIS

SYMPTOMS

Fever. Headache. Vomiting. Sore throat. Pain and stiffness in the back and neck. Drowsiness. In NON-PARALYTIC POLIO, fever usually lasts about 7 days and stiffness fades in 3 to 5 days. In PARALYTIC POLIO, weakness or paralysis of the arms or legs begins 1 to 7 days after the first symptoms. In BULBAR POLIO, which affects swallowing and breathing muscles, difficulty in swallowing, breathing and speaking may occur in the first 3 days of illness. A contagious viral disease affecting the nervous system. The period of communicability is not known. The virus is spread from the throat of the carrier and from infected feces, and enters the body through the mouth and nose.

WHAT TO DO
- **Consult your physician.**
- No specific treatment. In mild cases, only bed rest for several days may be needed. In more severe cases, treatment may include hot moist packs, physical therapy and medication. For respiratory difficulties, a mechanical respirator can be life-saving.
- A preventive vaccine is available.

ROSEOLA

SYMPTOMS

Begin with: Fever of 103° to 104°F./39.4° to 40°C. After 3 to 4 days: Fever falls. Reddish-pink rash appears on the chest and abdomen. May also affect the face and extremities to some extent. During the rash the child feels well. After 1 or 2 days: The rash disappears. An acute disease of infants and young children, believed to be caused by a virus.

WHAT TO DO
- **Consult your physician.**
- There is no specific treatment, but sponge baths may be used to reduce high fever. No further treatment is usually needed once the temperature becomes normal and the rash appears.

SCARLET FEVER (Scarlatina)

SYMPTOMS

Begin with: Fever as high as 105°F./40.5°C. Sore throat. Headache. Vomiting. Neck gland swelling. Strawberry-colored tongue. On the second day: A pinkish-red flush appears on the skin. The flush lasts 4 to 10 days and may be mild or widespread. Caused by streptococcal bacteria. Contagious from 24 hours before symptoms to 2 to 3 weeks afterward.

WHAT TO DO
- **Consult your physician.**
- Antibiotic treatment is effective and can help forestall possible complications such as rheumatic fever, meningitis and encephalitis.

SUDDEN INFANT DEATH

SYMPTOMS

None. The death is completely unexpected and without prior warning. Affecting 10,000 infants a year in the U.S., sudden infant deaths occur most often in the third and fourth months of life, with higher incidence in premature infants and infants living in poverty. More boys than girls are affected. More cases occur in winter than summer. Almost all deaths take place during sleep. The cause is uncertain. In about 10 percent of the cases, autopsies show unsuspected heart or nervous system abnormality or evidence of severe infection.

WHAT TO DO
- Parents losing a child from sudden infant death are totally unprepared and overwhelmed by grief. Because no cause can be found, they tend to blame themselves. Difficult as it may be, they must try to overcome this needless guilt. Counseling from trained nurses and from other parents who have experienced and adjusted to the tragedy can be valuable.

WHOOPING COUGH

SYMPTOMS
Begin with: Running nose. Sneezing. Eye tearing.
Other signs of cold-like illness, but only rarely fever. Hacking cough at night which gradually begins to appear by day. After 10 to 14 days, the cough becomes paroxysmal. There may be half a dozen to a dozen or more quick coughs followed by the whoop, a hurried deep breath. A highly communicable disease caused by bacteria. Can occur at any age but is most common before 2 years. Transmission is usually through the air from an infected person. Coughing lasts 4 to 6 weeks. The disease can be transmitted for about 4 weeks after the symptoms first appear.

WHAT TO DO
- **Consult your physician.**
- Hospitalization may be needed for a seriously ill infant. Bed rest may not be required for an older child with only a mild illness.
- Severe vomiting may be treated with intravenous fluids. Antibiotics may be prescribed for any complicating bacterial infections such as pneumonia or middle ear infection.
- A preventive vaccine is available.

CIRCULATORY SYSTEM

ANEURYSM (Artery ballooning)

SYMPTOMS
If the aneurysm is in the abdomen: Agonizing, boring pain in the abdomen or back. If it is in the chest: Chest or back pain. Coughing. Labored breathing. Swallowing difficulty. If in addition to ballooning, the artery has a ruptured inner coat so that blood escapes between the layers or the artery wall, splitting or dissecting the wall: Severe chest pain, similar to that of a heart attack. Aneurysm in a thigh may produce: Visible swelling which can expand and contract with the heartbeat. Most often affected by aneurysm is the aorta, the trunk-line artery which emerges from the heart and passes through the chest and abdomen. May be associated with artery hardening. Often accompanied by high blood pressure.

WHAT TO DO
- **Consult your physician.**
- Small at first, an aneurysm tends to increase in size with time until it may rupture, spilling blood. To keep this from happening, preventive surgery in advance of rupture may be recommended. The diseased section of artery is removed and replaced with a prosthetic graft. In some cases, medical treatment, including medication to bring down elevated blood pressure, may be prescribed.

ANGINA PECTORIS

SYMPTOMS
Pain behind the breastbone in the center of chest, usually brought on by exertion. The pain may spread in various ways — to the left shoulder, down inside the left arm, to the fingers; straight through into the back; or into the throat, jaw and teeth, and down the right arm. Pain subsides when activity stops. If it continues, may indicate heart attack. Caused by a coronary artery disease in which the fatty deposits in the arteries feeding the heart muscle reduce circulation.

WHAT TO DO
- **Consult your physician.**
- Nitroglycerin and other drugs can be used to cut short or even avoid angina attacks. If these fail to help, surgery to bypass diseased portions of the coronary arteries is very often successful.
- Treatment is also needed for the underlying coronary artery disease. Factors involved in the disease such as

high blood pressure, smoking and excess weight will have to be corrected.

ARTERIOSCLEROSIS / ATHEROSCLEROSIS

SYMPTOMS

May produce the chest pain of angina pectoris or coronary thrombosis; see ANGINA PECTORIS and CORONARY THROMBOSIS. May affect the leg arteries, causing pain on walking or even at rest. ARTERIOSCLEROSIS (hardening of the arteries) is an overall term which includes atherosclerosis. In **ATHEROSCLEROSIS,** deposits form on the inner lining of the arteries, narrowing the passageway for blood. It is the most prevalent artery disease.

WHAT TO DO

- **Consult your physician.**
- It may be extremely helpful to correct certain factors that are thought to increase the risk of arterio-atherosclerosis and its acceleration. Those factors include lack of exercise, excess weight, cigarette smoking, high levels of cholesterol and triglycerides (fats) in the blood, high blood pressure, uncontrolled diabetes and poor thyroid functioning.
- Consulting a nutritionist can be helpful.

ATRIAL FIBRILLATION

SYMPTOMS

Occasional irregular pulse. Feeling of fluttering in the chest. Pallor. Nausea. Weakness. Near-fainting. Light-headedness. Fatigue. An abnormally rapid rhythm of the atria, the two upper, blood-receiving chambers of the heart. May occur with coronary heart disease, heart attack, rheumatic heart disease, excessive thyroid gland functioning. Sometimes afflicts a normal heart.

WHAT TO DO

- **Consult your physician.**
- Treatment is aimed at reestablishing and maintaining normal heart rhythm. Medication may be prescribed. In some cases unresponsive to medication, electric stimulation of the heart may be used to reestablish normal rhythm.

CARDIAC NEUROSIS

SYMPTOMS

May include: Vague chest pain. Shortness of breath. Palpitations. Headache. Fatigue. Anxiety. Apprehensiveness. Flushing. Cold hands and feet. Also called "soldier's heart" and "functional heart trouble," cardiac neurosis involves no actual physical disease. May be

triggered by stress of battle or daily life. Sometimes it is a response to the heart attack death of a friend or family member.

WHAT TO DO

- **Consult your physician.**
- Cardiac neurosis is not to be dismissed lightly. Thorough examination and tests are needed to rule out any real heart trouble — and provide reassurance to the patient.

CONGENITAL HEART DISORDERS

SYMPTOMS

Some disorders may include: Blue appearance (cyanosis) in infancy. Later symptoms may include: Abnormal heart rate. Breathlessness. Abnormal heart sounds. Easy fatigue. Failure to grow properly. In some cases, there are no obvious symptoms until adolescence or adulthood, but the disorder may be detected earlier during a routine medical examination. Congenital heart disorders are present at birth in about 8 of every 1,000 children. They include abnormal openings in the interior walls of the heart, heart valve defects and narrowing of the aorta, the great trunk-line artery.

WHAT TO DO

- **Consult your physician.** Disorders can be diagnosed by expert physical examination, electrocardiograph and other tests.
- Treatment is usually surgical repair, which is highly successful in most cases.

CORONARY THROMBOSIS (Heart attack)

SYMPTOMS

Chest pain that may range from a feeling of pressure to a sensation of crushing. (Unlike angina chest pain, it does not stop with rest or nitroglycerin.) Great anxiety. Ashen face. Cold sweats. Shortness of breath. Often: Retching. Belching. Vomiting. May be preceded by a history of angina pectoris (see **ANGINA PECTORIS**), but can also appear suddenly, without prior symptoms. Results from the formation of a clot (thrombus) in an already-diseased (atherosclerotic) heart-feeding coronary artery.

WHAT TO DO

- **Seek medical aid immediately at the first suspicion of a heart attack. Summon a physician or emergency squad or get the person to a hospital emergency room. Cancel all doubts about acting; better safe than dead.**
- Treatment may include medication, oxygen and other measures to help the heart and to overcome or prevent potentially serious abnormal rhythms. (When left un-

treated, abnormal rhythms are a frequent cause of heart attack death.)

ENDOCARDITIS

SYMPTOMS

Low-grade fever (seldom over 102°F./38.9°C.), which may be irregular or sustained. Other symptoms may include: Chills. Malaise. Joint pains. Blotches on the palms and soles. Small red or purplish spots over much of the body. Enlarged, painful spleen. Fatigue. Appetite loss. Anemia. Chest pain may develop later. A bacterial infection of the heart lining. Often follows a dental procedure or injection of narcotics, especially but not only in people with already-damaged heart valves.

WHAT TO DO

- **Consult your physician immediately.** Unless treated properly, may be fatal.
- Treatment usually requires bed rest and antibiotics, administered for a month or more. The particular antibiotic used is determined by the infecting organisms and their sensitivity to it. Treatment may also be needed for anemia and may include transfusion if the anemia is severe.

EXTRA HEARTBEAT
(Premature or skipped beat)

SYMPTOMS

Feeling of an extra or a skipped heartbeat. Not accompanied by pain. The sensation may seem like a flutter in the chest. Can be brought on by excessive thyroid function or heart disease but commonly results from tension, fatigue, coffee or tea, smoking.

WHAT TO DO

- **Consult your physician.**
- Treatment will be directed at the thyroid or heart problem, if one is present. Otherwise, reassurance that there is nothing wrong with the heart may be enough. If necessary, medication may be prescribed.

HEART BLOCK

SYMPTOMS

Dizziness. Near-fainting. Sometimes: A palpitation and flutter in the chest. Rarely: Fainting. Convulsions. Involves slowing or interruption of the electrical activity that governs the work of the pumping chambers of the heart. May occur in chronic heart disease or sometimes as a result of overdoses of heart drugs.

WHAT TO DO

- **Consult your physician.**

- If drug overdosage is the cause, the condition will be corrected when the dosage is changed. Otherwise, a pacemaker — an electronic device that automatically controls the heartbeat — may be implanted surgically, allowing a normal life.

HEART FAILURE
(Congestive heart failure)

SYMPTOMS

Begin with: Gradual, progressive energy loss. Increasing breathing difficulty on exertion. Ankle swelling. Followed by: Labored breathing at rest. Other symptoms may include: Nausea. Appetite loss. Abdominal pain. Bluish color. In the elderly: Mental confusion. In congestive heart failure, the heart pumps out blood less efficiently, impairing the blood flow to the body tissues and allowing congestion in the lungs and circulation. May result from various types of heart disease, inflammation of the sac enclosing the heart (pericarditis), low thyroid function (hypothyroidism).

WHAT TO DO

- **Consult your physician.**
- Treatment includes finding and overcoming the underlying problem. Meanwhile, medication may be used to help the heart pump more effectively, and salt restriction and drugs may be prescribed to reduce fluid retention and congestion. If necessary, oxygen may be administered.

HIGH BLOOD PRESSURE
(Hypertension)

SYMPTOMS

None in the early stages. Later symptoms may include one or more of the following: Headache. Dizziness. Palpitation. Insomnia. Weakness. When uncontrolled for long periods may cause: Heart enlargement. Chest pain. Heart attack. Stroke. Eye changes. Kidney disturbances. Affecting more than 25 million Americans, almost half of whom aren't aware of it, hypertension can be a deadly disease. It is readily detected by a physician during routine examination.

WHAT TO DO

- **Consult your physician for periodic examination including blood pressure reading.** If hypertension is detected, treatment will be necessary.
- Treatment can be for the underlying cause (found in only about 10 percent of the cases), which may be a narrowing of the kidney artery or the aorta (the great trunkline artery), or a benign adrenal gland tumor. These are all curable by surgery. In most cases, treatment can control the blood pressure with weight reduction and decreased use of salt, sometimes combined with prescribed medication.

PERICARDITIS

SYMPTOMS

Dull or sharp chest pain under the breastbone. Fever. Chills. Weakness. Sometimes: Quick, shallow breathing. Nonproductive coughing. An inflammation of the sac enclosing the heart (pericardium). May follow pneumonia or a bone or other infection. Sometimes caused by tumor, rheumatic or other heart disease, or uremia.

WHAT TO DO

- **Consult your physician.**
- Treatment may include antibiotics and other medication, and in some cases withdrawal of fluid from the sac.

PERIPHERAL VASCULAR DISEASE

SYMPTOMS

Cramping leg pain on walking (intermittent claudication), which is relieved by rest. Other symptoms in the legs or arms may include: Coldness. Numbness. Tingling. Burning. Peripheral vascular (blood vessel) disease most commonly affects the legs. It may be due to obstruction resulting from atherosclerosis (fatty deposits). One form, **BUERGER'S DISEASE,** also known as thromboangiitis obliterans, is an inflammatory condition that roughens blood vessel inner walls and sometimes leads to clot formation. The cause is not entirely clear, but excessive smoking is believed to be a factor.

WHAT TO DO

- **Consult your physician.** Untreated, peripheral vascular disease can lead to gangrene and amputation.
- Treatment requires elimination of tobacco in all forms. Special foot care instructions may be given. The physician may prescribe medication to dilate the blood vessels (vasodilators) as well as special exercises to help stimulate circulation. When necessary, surgery may be recommended to bypass the obstruction.

PHLEBITIS
(Venous thrombosis, thrombophlebitis, phlebothrombosis, milk leg)

SYMPTOMS

Swelling in the leg. The leg feels heavy and painful. It takes on an unnatural whiteness. Involves a clot in a vein — either with little or no inflammation **(PHLEBOTHROMBOSIS),** or definite inflammation of a vein wall **(THROMBOPHLEBITIS, PHLEBITIS).** May occur because of injury, infection or the standstill of blood in the vein due to inactivity or bed rest. May follow surgery or pregnancy.

WHAT TO DO

- **Consult your physician.**
- Treatment may include bed rest with the leg elevated to aid the return flow of blood from the vein to the heart. Moist warm packs may also be used. An anticoagulant drug may be prescribed to help prevent further clotting. When the clot is in a superficial vein, bed rest may not be needed. Walking with an elastic support may be allowed, with intervals of leg elevation and applied heat.

PULMONARY EMBOLISM

SYMPTOMS

In some cases, breathlessness may be the only symptom. In other cases, symptoms may include: Chest pain. Fever. Coughing. Spitting of blood. A pulmonary embolism is a blood clot which usually forms in a deep leg vein, then breaks off and is carried in the bloodstream to a lung artery.

WHAT TO DO

- **Consult your physician.**
- If necessary, oxygen may be administered by face mask. The physician may prescribe a pain reliever and an anticoagulant drug. In some extreme cases, surgery may be required to remove the clot.

RAPID HEARTBEAT (Sinus tachycardia, paroxysmal tachycardia)

SYMPTOMS

The only symptom may be a fast, forceful beat of the heart, greater than 100 beats a minute, that comes on gradually, then slackens off (SINUS TACHYCARDIA). In other cases, an extremely rapid beat may develop suddenly, reaching 180 beats a minute or higher, and last for hours or days. It may disappear suddenly and then recur (PAROXYSMAL TACHYCARDIA). The very fast rate may be accompanied by: Nausea. Pallor. Weakness. Fainting. Possible causes of sinus tachycardia include emotional stress, exercise, infection, anemia, excessive thyroid functioning (hyperthyroidism). Paroxysmal tachycardia may occur in rheumatic or other heart disease but also in a normal heart and may stem from anxiety, fatigue, tobacco, tea or coffee.

WHAT TO DO

- **Consult your physician for a checkup and for treatment if necessary.**
- It is sometimes possible to interrupt paroxysmal tachycardia in one of several ways: lying down with the feet in the air, bending forward from the waist, exhaling or trying to inhale with the glottis (the opening between the vocal cords) closed, vomiting with the aid of warm bicarbonate of soda.

• When necessary, medication may be prescribed to restore a normal heart rate.

RHEUMATIC HEART DISEASE (Rheumatic fever)

SYMPTOMS

Rheumatic fever follows a strep tonsil, throat, ear or other infection, usually after 1 to 4 weeks. May begin with: Fever. Tiredness. Nosebleeds. Joint pain. Joint swelling. If a complicating heart inflammation develops, other symptoms may include: Rapid heartbeat. Heart murmur. Coughing. Chest pain. Shortness of breath. Rheumatic fever occurs most often among schoolchildren, rarely before age 4 or after 18. It is unclear why some persons with strep throats or other strep infections develop rheumatic fever. Family susceptibility seems to play a role, but it is not necessarily of paramount importance. Nor is it clear why some persons with rheumatic fever develop a heart complication which may sometimes, but not always, deform a heart valve.

WHAT TO DO

• **Consult your physician.**
• **Treatment requires bed rest.** Depending upon the severity, medication may be prescribed.
• After the acute attack is over, an antibiotic may be prescribed on a regular basis to help prevent further attacks. (Further attacks tend to increase the liklihood of heart damage.)
• In case of serious heart valve damage, corrective surgery may be recommended.

SHOCK

SYMPTOMS

Cold, moist, often bluish hands and feet. Weak and racing pulse. Falling blood pressure. Other symptoms may include: Confusion and anxiety, followed by lethargy. Nausea. Sweating. Chest pain. Breathing difficulty. A POTENTIALLY GRAVE EMERGENCY, medical shock — unrelated to electrical shock — involves a disruption of circulation, with blood pressure falling so low that the blood may not get to the vital tissues. It can develop after severe injury, surgery, hemorrhage, dehydration, heart attack, severe infection, poisoning, drug reaction.

WHAT TO DO

• **Seek medical aid immediately. If possible, call for an ambulance.**
• Meanwhile, to help the blood flow to the brain, keep the person lying down on his back, with his head lower than the rest of his body. Check his airway for possible obstruction; remove any mucus or vomit. Cover the person to keep him warm. Stop any bleeding with

pressure or a bandage; see **BLEEDING: CUTS & WOUNDS** in Part One. If breathing has stopped, start resuscitation; see **BREATHING: ARTIFICIAL RESPIRATION** in Part One. If he is unconscious and vomiting, place him on his side to help prevent breathing in vomit. When definitive medical treatment becomes available, it may include transfusion, intravenous fluids, therapy for the cause of the shock.

SLOW HEARTBEAT (Sinus bradycardia)

SYMPTOMS

If slowing is not severe, there are no symptoms. If it is very severe, symptoms may include: Fainting. Convulsions. Generally, slow heartbeat — less than 60 beats a minute — indicates good health. It is common in athletes and often occurs normally in sleep. Rates of 40 to 60 beats a minute usually produce no symptoms. Slower rates may cause fatigue and decreased exercise tolerance. Rates below 30 may require treatment. Sometimes may be caused by low thyroid function, illness, drug intoxication.

WHAT TO DO

• **Consult your physician if symptoms occur.** If necessary, medication may be prescribed.

STROKE

SYMPTOMS

Depending upon the brain area affected, symptoms may include: Paralysis of one side of the body. Speech disturbance. Defective vision. Coma. Confusion. Headache. Stroke involves destruction of an area of the brain tissue due to an interruption of the blood supply to that area. It may be caused by rupture of a vessel and bleeding within the cranium, spasm or contraction of a vessel, or blockage by a clot that either formed in the vessel or traveled there from elsewhere in the body. High blood pressure is a major factor. Atherosclerotic narrowing of arteries in the brain as well as elsewhere in the body is common.

NOTE: In many cases, before a major stroke occurs, there are warning signals, **LITTLE STROKES. The symptoms of little strokes include: Fleeting episodes of dizziness. Burning or tingling sensations. Weakness of one side of the body. Confusion. Visual disturbances.** The symptoms last from 2 or 3 minutes to 30 minutes.

WHAT TO DO

• **For a major stroke, seek medical aid immediately.** Immediate treatment and skilled nursing care are essential. During convalescence, physiotherapy (for the paralysis) and speech therapy may be needed.
• **For little strokes, consult your physician without delay.** These warning signals should not be neglected.

Often, they can be traced to an artery blockage which can be treated by surgery before a major stroke occurs.

VARICOSE VEINS

SYMPTOMS

Swollen, distended and knotted veins, especially in the legs. In some cases: Leg fatigue. Leg soreness. May develop from sluggish blood flow or defective valves in the veins. Prolonged standing or sitting without movement may contribute to the development since blood return from the legs is helped by leg muscle activity. Varicosities (which may be temporary) may develop in pregnancy if the uterus presses against veins returning from the legs, inducing back pressures that interfere with free blood flow. Some recent studies suggest that constipation and straining at stool may be important factors in developing varicose veins because of the resultant back pressure.

WHAT TO DO

• In mild cases, bathing the legs in warm water may help by aiding the blood flow. Several rest periods each day, with the feet above the body, may also encourage the flow of blood. Elasticized stockings can be helpful. To combat constipation, it may be advisable to increase the fiber in the diet through whole grain cereals, bran, vegetables and fruits. Consulting a nutritionist can be helpful.
• **For severe cases, consult your physician.** Surgery may be recommended to tie off and remove a varicosed vein, or a hardening solution may be injected.

VENTRICULAR FIBRILLATION

SYMPTOMS

Fainting. Total collapse. No pulse. The distinct heartbeat is replaced by a useless twitching of the heart, which is incapable of pumping blood. May result from heart attack, drug overdose or electric shock. **A GRAVE EMERGENCY.** Death is imminent.

WHAT TO DO

• **Seek medical aid immediately. If possible, call an ambulance or rescue team.** Most hospitals and many ambulances and rescue teams have a defibrillator, an electrical device to shock the heart back to its normal rhythm through electrodes placed on the chest.
• Until help arrives, begin CPR (cardiopulmonary resuscitation); see **HEART FAILURE** in Part One.

DIGESTIVE SYSTEM: ANUS

ANAL FISSURE

SYMPTOMS

Painful spasm or contraction of the anal sphincter (control muscle). Especially intense pain on defecation. A small crack or tear in the mucous membrane of the rectum or the skin around the anus which deepens and becomes inflamed. Usually results from the passage of large hard stools.

WHAT TO DO

• **Consult your physician.** Cure is often possible in 2 to 3 weeks.
• Treatment may include low-residue diet, stool softener, anesthetic ointment used before and after defecation. Sitting in a warm tub immediately after defecation often helps relax the spasm. If a fissure becomes chronic, it may be repaired by relatively minor surgery.

ANAL FISTULA

SYMPTOMS

Pus discharge near the anus. Skin irritation. Often with repeated abscess formation. An abnormal tunnel leading from inside the rectum to the outside skin. Often results from an infection in the anal or rectal wall, which leads to the formation of an abscess that breaks the skin near the anal opening and forms a tunnel or fistula.

WHAT TO DO

• **Consult your physician.**
• Surgical repair is required. A fistula does not heal without medical attention.

ANAL PRURITUS (Itching)

SYMPTOMS

Chronic severe itching in the anal area. Worsens at night. Aggravated by scratching and heat. Possible causes include poor anal hygiene, minor injury from defecation, irritating soaps and clothing, anal fissure, anal fistula, hemorrhoids, infectious agents, intestinal parasites (especially pinworms), allergies, jaundice, diabetes, uremia and lymphoma.

WHAT TO DO

• **Consult your physician.** He will have to search for the cause before he can correct the condition.

• Treatment may include avoidance of scratching and frequent use of talc or dusting powder after gentle drying with cotton or tissue. Medication may be prescribed to provide relief. Anesthetic or other ointments are not advisable since they may macerate the skin and make it more prone to injury.

ANORECTAL ABSCESS

SYMPTOMS

Red swelling in the anal area. Often makes walking, sitting or defecation painful. May start as an infection of the anal or rectal glands or be associated with an anal fissure or an intestinal disease such as regional enteritis or ulcerative colitis.

WHAT TO DO

• **Consult your physician.**
• Incision and drainage are required. Antibiotics may be prescribed when the infection is widespread.

HEMORRHOIDS (Piles)

SYMPTOMS

If hemorrhoids are EXTERNAL (outside the rectum) symptoms may be limited to: Mild itching. Some discomfort during defecation. If hemorrhoids are INTERNAL (inside the rectum), symptoms may include: Rectal fullness. Bleeding. Quite painful defecation. Hemorrhoids are enlarged varicose veins in the rectal area. May result from increased pressure caused by pregnancy, obesity, chronic coughing or sneezing, constipation and straining at stool, abdominal tumors.

WHAT TO DO

• Small hemorrhoids causing no more than occasional slight bleeding may need no treatment other than avoiding constipation and straining at stool. For constipation, it may be helpful to increase the fiber in the diet through whole meal breads, whole grain cereals, bran, vegetables and fruit. Consulting a nutritionist can be helpful.
• **For other hemorrhoids, consult your physician.** Treatment may include heat applications, cold compresses, sitting in warm baths, medicated ointment or suppositories. In some cases, uncomplicated bleeding internal hemorrhoids may be treated by injection. Surgical removal may not be required unless the bleeding is severe, the hemorrhoids protrude in a large mass or the anal itching is unbearable. New removal techniques include applying special rubber bands to the hemorrhoids to cause them to slough off.

PROCTITIS

SYMPTOMS

Rectal discomfort. Repeated urge to move the bowels. Painful diarrhea. Blood, pus and mucus in stools. An inflammation of the mucous membrane lining the rectum. Most commonly caused by the intestinal disorders of regional enteritis and ulcerative colitis. May also stem from infection, injury, some drugs.

WHAT TO DO

• **Consult your physician.**
• If possible, the specific underlying cause must be treated. Treatment may also include suppositories, retention enemas containing medication, and in some cases stool softeners, spasm-reducing drugs and medication for the diarrhea.

DIGESTIVE SYSTEM: ESOPHAGUS

ACHALASIA (Cardiospasm)

SYMPTOMS

Progressively increasing difficulty in swallowing both solids and liquids. In some cases, nightly regurgitation of undigested food occurs, with the risk of being inhaled into the lungs, causing lung abscess or pneumonia. There may also be chest pain. Failure of the lower end of the esophagus to relax normally so that food and drink can pass freely into the stomach. The cause is unknown.

WHAT TO DO

• **Consult your physician.**
• Dilation of the lower esophagus with an instrument is often successful. (It produces good results in 80 percent of the patients.) When this fails, surgery is usually successful.

BENIGN TUMOR OF THE ESOPHAGUS

SYMPTOMS

Swallowing difficulty. Often with a feeling of fullness or pressure. The tumor is usually small and generally remains so, rarely exceeding the size of a small marble. The cause is unknown.

WHAT TO DO

• **Consult your physician.**
• Surgery may be recommended.

ESOPHAGITIS

SYMPTOMS

Burning pain behind the breastbone. Swallowing difficulty. Heartburn. Inflammation of the lining of the esophagus. May result from infection, upsurge (reflux) of acid from the stomach, smoking, irritation from some foods, drugs.

WHAT TO DO

- **Consult your physician.**
- Treatment may include bland diet, avoidance of reclining soon after meals.

FOREIGN BODY IN THE ESOPHAGUS

SYMPTOMS

Sensation of something stuck in the gullet. If the esophagus has perforated or ruptured: Chest pains. Breathlessness. Occurs in adults as well as children from accidentally swallowing fish, poultry or meat bones or other foreign objects, sometimes even dentures.

WHAT TO DO

- **Seek medical aid immediately. If your physician isn't available, go to an emergency room.**
- If there is no perforation, the object often can be removed with instruments. In some cases, surgery may be recommended.
- Perforation can be an emergency, requiring expeditious surgical closure and antibiotics to avoid serious infection.

GLOBUS HYSTERICUS

SYMPTOMS

Sensation of a lump in the throat that is unrelated to swallowing. Although the sensation seems real enough, there is no lump and no impairment of the food passage. Often occurs in association with grief and other emotional problems.

WHAT TO DO

- **Consult your physician.** Any possible physical cause must be ruled out.
- Reassurance from a thorough examination often helps. If it doesn't, psychiatric aid may be needed.

ULCER OF THE ESOPHAGUS

SYMPTOMS

Severe pain after eating. The pain starts under the breastbone, and may radiate to the back. Heartburn. Sometimes: Belching of acid. Appetite loss. Weight loss. Ulcer of the esophagus resembles a peptic (stomach or duodenal) ulcer. The basic cause is not clear.

WHAT TO DO

- **Consult your physician.**
- Treatment may include a bland diet for a time, followed by elimination of any foods that have been found to cause distress. Medication may also be prescribed.

ZENKER'S DIVERTICULUM OF THE ESOPHAGUS

SYMPTOMS

Difficulty in swallowing after the first few bites of food. Sometimes, a gurgling noise during eating or drinking. On bending or lying down, food may be regurgitated. The diverticulum is an outpouching of the esophagus lining, forming a pocket which sometimes fills with food, enlarges and causes swallowing difficulty.

WHAT TO DO

- **Consult your physician.**
- For a small pouch, no treatment may be needed. Sometimes, for a larger pouch, leaning to the side while eating may help avoid getting food into the pocket. For severe swallowing difficulty, surgical correction may be recommended.

DIGESTIVE SYSTEM: INTESTINES

APPENDICITIS

SYMPTOMS

Nausea. Abdominal pain. Appetite loss. Sometimes: Fever. Constipation. Diarrhea. The pain begins in the navel area, then shifts to the right lower quarter of the abdomen. It may be increased by coughing, sneezing, movement. Inflammation of the appendix, a hollow, 2-1/2- to 3-1/2-inch structure at the site where the large and small intestines join. Inflammation may develop when the appendix becomes obstructed by fecal material (occasionally by worms), allowing multiplication of bacteria.

WHAT TO DO

- **Consult your physician immediately.** Expert diagnosis is needed including a physical examination and a white blood cell count.

- Surgical removal of the appendix may be recommended.

CELIAC DISEASE

Flatulence. Stools that are large, frothy, pale, foul-smelling and fatty. Other symptoms may include: Abdominal distention. Muscle wasting and weakness. Vomiting. Failure to thrive. A relatively uncommon childhood disease — the adult form is called sprue — celiac involves an intolerance of gluten (the protein of wheat and rye), thought to be linked with hereditary influences. This intolerance causes abnormal changes in the small intestine lining and impaired absorption of nutrients. The disease usually begins after 6 months of age but may sometimes appear much later, even in adulthood.

WHAT TO DO

- **Consult your physician.**
- Proper diet is essential in treatment. It should be well-balanced, high in calories and protein, normal in fat, and exclude all cereal grains except rice and corn. Food labels must be inspected to eliminate any foods containing wheat, rye, barley and oat proteins. Supplements of iron, calcium and B and other vitamins may be needed to overcome any deficiencies. Consulting a nutritionist can be helpful.

CONSTIPATION

SYMPTOMS

Difficult or infrequent passage of stools. May sometimes be caused by organic problems such as intestinal obstruction, diverticulitis, gastrointestinal cancer, infections, thyroid or other gland disorders. Most often, however, the problem lies with poor bowel habits, poor diet or laxative or enema abuse.

WHAT TO DO

- For chronic constipation, all that may be needed is a change in diet, with increased intake of high fiber foods such as whole grain cereals, bran, fruits, vegetables and plenty of water. Consulting a nutritionist can be helpful. Frequent use of laxatives or enemas should be stopped. A regular toilet time should be established.
- **Consult your physician** for suddenly appearing constipation which could possibly have an organic cause.

CONSTIPATION, IMAGINARY

SYMPTOMS

Failure to have a daily bowel movement. Excessive concern with the bowels. Often: Heavy reliance on laxatives and enemas.

WHAT TO DO

- It is important to recognize that daily bowel movements are not required for health. It can be quite normal for some people to have a movement no more than once every two or three days. As long as there are no symptoms (except for possible needless anxiety), the lack of a daily movement should be of no concern.

INTESTINAL OBSTRUCTION

SYMPTOMS

Vary with obstruction site and degree. In COMPLETE SMALL INTESTINE OBSTRUCTION, symptoms include: Intermittent severe cramplike pain in the navel area. Vomiting becoming fecal in character. No passage of gas. No bowel movement. With PARTIAL SMALL INTESTINE OBSTRUCTION, symptoms are similar but less severe and diarrhea may occur. In COMPLETE LARGE INTESTINE (COLON) OBSTRUCTION, symptoms include: Similar pain. Infrequent vomiting. Gradual abdominal distention. In PARTIAL COLON OBSTRUCTION, symptoms include: Intermittent cramps low in the abdomen. Constipation or constipation alternating with diarrhea. Obstructions have many possible causes, including adhesions after surgery, hernia, tumor pressure, foreign bodies, impacted feces, telescoping of one part of the bowel into another (intussusception), twisting of a loop of intestine (volvulus), a clot in a bowel artery or vein, failure of bowel contractions (paralytic ileus) after surgery or with gallstones, kidney stones, peritonitis.

WHAT TO DO

- **Consult your physician.**
- Suction applied through a stomach tube will often remove intestinal contents regurgitated into the stomach. If this suction isn't enough, a long intestinal tube may be inserted. The intestinal tube is often effective in overcoming partial obstruction or paralytic ileus. In complete obstruction, surgery may be recommended.

IRRITABLE COLON
(Spastic colon, mucous colitis)

SYMPTOMS

Vary greatly. Episodes may last days, weeks or months. Symptoms may include one or more of the following: Abdominal pain (sharp or dull, on the right side or the left) often relieved by bowel movement or flatus passage. Constipation or constipation alternating with diarrhea. Mucus in the stools. Nausea. Heartburn. Belching. Headache. Weakness. Usually begins in early adult life. A very common problem often associated with stress. May affect most people to a degree at some time, some people recurrently.

WHAT TO DO

- **Consult your physician.** A careful medical checkup is

important to rule out other problems such as ulcerative colitis or diverticulitis.
- Treatment may include reassurance, addition of unprocessed bran to the diet, regular exercise, medication.

MALABSORPTION SYNDROME

SYMPTOMS

Vary. May include one or more of the following: Diarrhea. Weakness. Weight loss. Poor appetite. Protruberant abdomen. Pallor. Tendency to bleed. Sore tongue. Muscle cramps. Skin scaling. Bone pain. Symptoms result from impaired absorption of nutrients in the small intestine. Possible causes include parasitic disease, gland disorder, drug-induced malabsorption. For the two most important underlying problems, see **SPRUE** and **CELIAC DISEASE.**

WHAT TO DO

- **Consult your physician.**
- Thorough examination and laboratory studies, including stool checks, are needed to pinpoint and treat the cause.

MECKEL'S DIVERTICULUM

SYMPTOMS

May include any or many of the symptoms of appendicitis; see APPENDICITIS. The diverticulum is a sac attached to the small intestine, present in the fetus but normally disappearing after birth. In 1 to 2 percent of people, it remains, serving no purpose, and may at some point, like the appendix, become impacted with fecal material and become infected.

WHAT TO DO

- **Consult your physician.**
- Treatment is surgical.

MEGACOLON

SYMPTOMS

Severe constipation. Abdominal distention. Vomiting. Appetite loss. Occurs in some infants because of a congenital defect, a lack of nerve cells in a portion of the colon that prevents normal movement of fecal matter. This **CONGENITAL** form is called Hirschsprung's disease. Another form that is **ACQUIRED** affects older, usually mentally ill children, who refuse to try to defecate.

WHAT TO DO

- **Consult your physician.**
- Surgical treatment may be recommended for

Hirschsprung's disease, eliminating the affected part of the colon and connecting the remaining healthy parts. In most cases, this will bring about good bowel control.
- For acquired megacolon, psychiatric treatment is recommended along with use of laxatives and enemas until bowel training succeeds.

PERITONITIS

SYMPTOMS

Severe, constant, prostrating abdominal pain, exacerbated by movement. Fever. Chills. Nausea. Vomiting. Sometimes: Diarrhea. An acute inflammation of the membrane (peritoneum) lining the abdominal cavity and covering the abdominal organs. Can be caused by infection or irritation from organisms or chemicals penetrating to the peritoneum as a result of a burst appendix, perforated ulcer or ruptured gallbladder, spleen or bladder.

WHAT TO DO

- **Consult your physician immediately.** Immediate treatment is urgent.
- Antibiotic therapy, along with agents to relieve pain, may precede surgical repair.

REGIONAL ENTERITIS
(Crohn's disease, ileitis)

SYMPTOMS

Chronic diarrhea. Abdominal pain. Fever. Appetite loss. Weight loss. Abdominal mass. Other symptoms may include: Arthritis. Repeated episodes of severe intestinal colic. An inflammation of unknown cause, usually of the lower ileum, the last portion of the small intestine. Sometimes affects other areas of the bowel.

WHAT TO DO

- **Consult your physician.**
- No specific treatment is available. Diet, antibiotics and other medication may be prescribed to relieve the symptoms. In some cases, surgery is recommended.

SPRUE (Adult celiac disease)

SYMPTOMS

Diarrhea with light-colored, frothy, fatty, malodorous stools. Other symptoms may include: Appetite loss. Weight loss. Weakness. Pallor. Brown pigmentation of the skin. Abdominal distension. A chronic disease of unknown cause that impairs the absorption of fats and some vitamins. Occurs in adults over 30.

- **Consult your physician.**
- Treatment includes vitamin and mineral supplements and a well-balanced diet that excludes all cereal grains except rice and corn (no wheat, barley, rye or oat proteins). Consulting a nutritionist can be helpful.

ULCERATIVE COLITIS

SYMPTOMS

Episodes of diarrhea (a dozen or more movements a day). Often with: Abdominal cramps. Fever. Blood and mucus in stools. Malaise. Anemia. Appetite loss. Weight loss. In severe cases, symptoms may include: Stools consisting almost entirely of blood and pus. Of unknown cause, the disease inflames and ulcerates the colon. It may affect any age but most often begins between 15 and 40. There is some familial tendency toward it.

WHAT TO DO

- **Consult your physician.**
- About 10 percent of patients recover completely after one attack, but the disease is usually chronic. The treatment depends upon the severity. It may include such measures as: medication to reduce cramps and stool frequency, high-protein high-calorie diet, antibiotics or other antibacterials, blood transfusion if anemia is severe. If medical measures fail, surgical removal of the affected portion of the colon may be recommended.

DIGESTIVE SYSTEM: STOMACH

ACUTE GASTROENTERITIS (Including food poisoning)

SYMPTOMS

Nausea. Vomiting. Cramps. Gas sounds (rumblings). Diarrhea. An inflammation of the stomach and intestinal lining. May be caused by intestinal "flu" virus, excessive alcohol intake, food poisoning, cathartics, drugs (such as aspirin and related compounds, colchicine, quinacrine), or by infections such as amebic dysentery and typhoid fever. **FOOD INFECTION GASTROENTERITIS,** caused by food contaminated with salmonella bacteria, usually appears 6 to 48 hours after ingestion and may produce additional symptoms of headache and muscle aches. **STAPHYLOCOCCUS TOXIN GASTROENTERITIS,** the most common type of food poisoning, is caused by foods (such as custards, cream-filled pastries, milk, fish, processed meat) contaminated with a toxin or poison formed by staph bacteria. It occurs within 2 to 4 hours and produces symptoms similar to those of food infection gastroenteritis.

WHAT TO DO

- Bed rest is indicated. No food or drink should be consumed until the nausea and vomiting disappear; then light fluids (tea, broth, cereal, bouillon with salt) may be taken. When these are well tolerated, other foods may be gradually added.
- **Consult your physician** if symptoms are very severe and vomiting persists. Medication to control vomiting and, if necessary, intravenous fluids to prevent dehydration may be prescribed. Except in rare cases, antibiotic treatment may not be needed.

GASTRITIS (Acute and chronic)

SYMPTOMS

Depend upon the form of gastritis (inflammation of the lining of the stomach). **Symptoms of ACUTE EROSIVE GASTRITIS: Nausea. Vomiting (sometimes of blood). Dizziness. Headache. Abdominal pressure. Appetite loss.** Causes include drugs (especially aspirin), excessive alcohol intake, hot spicy foods, allergic sensitivity to some foods, food poisoning, viral and other acute illness. **Symptoms of ACUTE CORROSIVE GASTRITIS: Possible corrosion of the lips, tongue, mouth and throat. Inflamed esophagus with pain and swallowing difficulty. Severe stomach pain. Vomiting of blood. Bluish color. Collapse.** May be caused by swallowing strong acid or alkali, heavy metal salt, iodine or potassium permanganate. **Symptoms of CHRONIC GASTRITIS may include: Mild nausea. Discomfort on eating. Burning sensation over the stomach area.** The cause is sometimes unknown but chronic gastritis may develop with pernicious anemia, diabetes, chronic aspirin use, stomach cancer or thyroid, adrenal or pituitary gland disorders.

WHAT TO DO

- **Consult your physician.**
- For acute erosive gastritis, little treatment may be needed since the stomach lining is usually renewed every 36 hours. But the cause should be determined and removed. Medication for nausea and vomiting may be prescribed.
- For acute corrosive gastritis, prompt treatment, often in a hospital, is needed. May include antidotes, drugs to induce vomiting and a stomach tube to remove the causative material.

- For chronic gastritis, any underlying disease should be corrected. Avoiding foods that aggravate the symptoms may help. Antacids may be prescribed.

INDIGESTION (Dyspepsia)

SYMPTOMS

During or after a meal, may include: Nausea. Heartburn. Upper abdominal pain. Flatulence. Belching. Feelings of fullness and stomach distention. Can be caused by stomach or intestinal disease or a disease elsewhere in the body, but commonly involves no organic disorder. Often stems from overeating, rapid eating, eating during emotional upsets, excessive air swallowing, smoking, poorly prepared foods, high-fat foods, gas-forming vegetables such as beans, cabbage, onions and turnips.

WHAT TO DO

- **Consult your physician.**
- If there is no underlying organic disorder, treatment may include a balanced diet, eating moderate amounts unhurriedly in a relaxed environment, not smoking before eating and avoiding any foods that contribute to the symptoms. Consulting a nutritionist can be helpful.

PANCREATITIS (Acute and chronic)

SYMPTOMS

In the ACUTE form: Severe, steady, boring abdominal pain. (It is often sharpest about the stomach area, extends to the back and chest and is relieved in many cases by sitting up.) Fever. Nausea. Vomiting. An acute inflammation of the pancreas. May follow injury, abdominal surgery, penetrating peptic ulcer, infectious disease, pregnancy, use of some drugs (corticosteroids, diuretics). **In the CHRONIC form: Abdominal pain. (It may be mild or severe, constant or intermittent and begins in the stomach area, then spreads to the back and left shoulder.) Other symptoms may include: Jaundice (yellowed skin).** Has the same causes as the acute form. Most common predisposing factor: excessive alcohol intake. Gallstones are sometimes involved.

WHAT TO DO

- **Consult your physician.**
- Treatment for acute pancreatitis may include suction of the stomach by tube to reduce distention and minimize stimulation of the pancreas, atropine to reduce pancreatic secretion, pain-relieving agents, antibiotics if infection develops. If there is an underlying disease, it will also have to be treated.
- Chronic pancreatitis receives similar treatment. If pain does not yield to medication, partial removal of the pancreas may be recommended. Alcohol is forbidden. Sometimes a special diet and vitamin and mineral supplements are also prescribed. Consulting a nutritionist can be helpful.

PEPTIC ULCER
(And ulcer complications)

SYMPTOMS

Pain in the upper abdomen over the stomach region. (It is usually mild or only moderately severe and described as burning, gnawing or aching.) Soreness. Empty feeling. Hunger. In DUODENAL ULCER (first portion of the intestine), pain first appears in midmorning, is relieved by food or antacid, recurs an hour or so after eating. Pain may also awaken the patient at night. In GASTRIC (STOMACH) ULCER, eating may cause pain instead of relieving it. Peptic ulcer, an area of erosion, most often occurs in the duodenum. The cause is not fully understood but involves excessive acid secretion and an impaired ability of the stomach lining to protect itself.
NOTE: Possible complications: PERFORATION — a tear in the stomach or duodenal wall — sometimes occurs. Symptoms may include: Agonizing abdominal pain. Boardlike and tender abdomen over the ulcer site. Fever. Shallow breathing. Another complication, MASSIVE HEMORRHAGE, can lead to: Weakness. Faintness. Profuse sweating. Vomiting of blood. Tarry stools. A third complication, OBSTRUCTION OF THE STOMACH OUTLET INTO THE SMALL INTESTINE, may cause: Foul belching. Vomiting of previous meals.

WHAT TO DO

- **Consult your physician.**
- Definite diagnosis of an ulcer can be established by x-ray. Treatment can relieve symptoms within a few days and may help speed healing. Dietary changes and medication may be prescribed.
- **Perforation is a surgical emergency. The tear must be closed.**
- In a massive hemorrhage, if bleeding fails to stop within 24 hours, surgery may be recommended.
- Obstruction of the stomach outlet may be treated by medication for pain and vomiting, liquid feedings, suction through the nose. If the obstruction does not disappear, surgery may be recommended.

POSTGASTRECTOMY
("Dumping syndrome")

SYMPTOMS

Soon after eating: Weakness. Dizziness. Sweating. Nausea. Vomiting. Palpitations. Sometimes follows surgery for removal of part or all of the stomach.

WHAT TO DO

- **Consult your physician.**
- Treatment may include a high-protein diet, frequent small feedings of dry food, lying down after a large meal, little or no liquids during or soon after meals, medication.

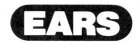

EARS

BOILS IN THE EAR CANAL

SYMPTOMS

Pain. Feeling of fullness in the ear. Impaired hearing. Neck and gland swelling. Boils, inflamed lumps with central cores, are caused by bacteria. They may develop in the ear alone or as part of an outbreak of boils elsewhere.

WHAT TO DO

• **Consult your physician.**
• A boil may be treated with medication, or it may be incised and the core removed.

CAULIFLOWER EAR

SYMPTOMS

Misshapen ear resulting from injury or blows. Caused by bleeding under the skin and clot formation, with possible damage to the ear cartilage.

WHAT TO DO

• **Consult your physician.**
• Treatment may require incision and removal of the clot, followed by splinting and a pressure dressing.

EUSTACHIAN TUBE OBSTRUCTION

SYMPTOMS

Pain. Feeling of fullness or pressure in the ear. Impaired hearing. Ringing in the ear. Dizziness. May result from enlarged adenoids blocking the eustachian tube opening in the throat, a common cold, allergy, tumor mass or fast descent in an airplane.

WHAT TO DO

• **Consult your physician** if symptoms persist.

EXTERNAL OTITIS (Swimmer's ear)

SYMPTOMS

Pain. Itching. An ear canal infection caused by contaminated water left in the ear.

WHAT TO DO

• **Consult your physician.** Although often dismissed as a minor matter, the infection sometimes can move inward and affect the hearing and balance.
• Treatment may include antibiotics, alcohol to dry the moisture, acetic acid to restore the protective acid mantle to the ear.

• Often can be prevented by thoroughly drying the canals after swimming, fanning the ear canal openings and shaking the head to remove any trapped water.

FUNGUS INFECTION OF EAR CANAL

SYMPTOMS

Severe itching. Some pain. Gray or black particles of fungi may be seen in the ear. Can result from inadequate ear hygiene or swimming in polluted water.

WHAT TO DO

• **Consult your physician.**

HEARING LOSS

SYMPTOMS

In CONDUCTIVE hearing loss (impaired transmission of sound through the ear canal and middle ear): The person still hears his own voice by conduction through the skull bones and tends to speak softly. In SENSORINEURAL loss (damage in the inner ear or the hearing nerve): The person hears his own voice only faintly and tends to speak loudly. Although he hears some sounds normally, he may not be able to make out high frequency sounds and sounds like p, k, t and hard g. Conductive loss may result from wax in the ear, water in the ear, blockage of the eustachian tube, boils in the ear and infections such as otitis media (middle ear infection) and mastoiditis. It often occurs because of otosclerosis, in which one of the tiny conducting bones in the middle ear becomes fixed in place and is no longer free to move and transmit sound. Sensorineural loss may result from long exposure to loud noise, injury, sensitivity to some drugs (such as aspirin, the antibiotic streptomycin) and as a complication of some diseases such as measles, mumps, meningitis, strep infections.

WHAT TO DO

• **Consult your physician.**
• Various tests can define the type of deafness and may be able to determine a correctable cause. Provided it is expertly prescribed and fitted, a hearing aid can be helpful. For otosclerosis, surgery can remove the defective bone and replace it with a plastic device or vein graft. In most cases, this will improve the hearing markedly or even restore it totally.

MASTOIDITIS

SYMPTOMS

Redness, swelling and tenderness over the mastoid

bone behind the ear. **Ear pain. Fever. Discharge from the ear canal.** An inflammation of the mastoid bone, most often caused by an untreated or inadequately treated middle ear infection. A disease to be taken seriously, since the mastoid bone is close to the brain; if not treated properly, the inflammation may lead to meningitis or a brain abscess.

WHAT TO DO
- Consult your physician.
- Antibiotic treatment, begun early, is usually effective. Surgery is not needed in most cases.

MENIÈRE'S DISEASE

SYMPTOMS

Recurring episodes of: Hearing loss. Ear ringing. Dizziness. Nausea. Vomiting. Sometimes: Eyeball oscillation (nystagmus). A disturbance of the inner ear, most often affecting one ear. The cause is unknown.

WHAT TO DO
- Consult your physician.
- Medication may be prescribed to help relieve symptoms. In severe cases, surgery may be recommended.

MOTION SICKNESS

SYMPTOMS

Nausea. Vomiting. Cold sweating. Pallor. Sometimes: Headache. Dizziness. Caused by excessive stimulation of the inner ear mechanisms by motion. Contributing causes include visual stimuli, such as a moving horizon, and emotional factors such as fear and anxiety.

WHAT TO DO
- Anyone susceptible to motion sickness should try to ride amidships or, in airplanes, over the wings, where there is least motion. A supine or semi-recumbent position often helps. Reading should be avoided.
- If taken before nausea and vomiting occur, anti-motion sickness drugs often help prevent sickness.

OTITIS MEDIA (Middle ear infection)

SYMPTOMS

Symptoms of ACUTE otitis media (inflammation of one or both ears) include: Earache. Feeling of fullness in the ear. Fever. Chills. Sometimes: Ear ringing. Impaired hearing. May be caused by organisms spreading to the middle ear from the nose and throat through the eustachian tubes or an eardrum injury. **Symptoms of CHRONIC CONGESTIVE otitis media: Gradual hearing loss. Ear ringing. Dizziness. Rarely: Pain.** May follow repeated attacks of acute otitis media or nose and throat infections affecting the eustachian tubes. **Symptoms of CHRONIC PURULENT otitis media: Discharge of pus from the**

ear. **Feeling of fullness in the ear. Impaired hearing. Low-grade fever. Ear ringing.** Usually proceded by acute otitis media or mastoiditis.

WHAT TO DO
- Consult your physician.
- For acute otitis media, treatment may include antibiotics, heat, antihistamines and decongestants to keep the eustachian tubes open and allow drainage from the middle ear. Sometimes an eardrum incision is needed.
- For chronic congestive otitis media, treatment may include inflation of the eustachian tube and temporary insertion of a plastic tube in the middle ear.
- For chronic purulent otitis media, treatment may include antibiotics by mouth, medicated ear drops, other local applications.

PERFORATED EARDRUM

SYMPTOMS

Severe ear pain. Hearing loss. Sometimes: Dizziness. Nausea. Vomiting. Blood in the ear canal. May result from a blow to the head, cleaning the ears with sharp objects, sometimes from pus accumulation during a middle ear infection.

WHAT TO DO
- Consult your physician.
- Small perforations often heal on their own. Larger ones may require surgical repair. Medication for pain may be prescribed.

SUDDEN DEAFNESS

SYMPTOMS

Profound hearing loss, usually in one ear, developing in a few hours or less. Sometimes: Ear ringing. Dizziness. Believed to be viral in origin.

WHAT TO DO
- Consult your physician.
- Treatment may include bed rest and prescribed medication.
- Dizziness usually disappears a few days after treatment. In most cases, hearing returns within 2 weeks.

VESTIBULAR NEURONITIS

SYMPTOMS

Sudden dizziness, first persistent, then paroxysmal. Believed to be an inflammation of a division of the hearing nerve produced by viruses. Often occurs in epidemics, especially among adolescents and young adults.

WHAT TO DO
- Consult your physician.
- The disorder is benign. The attacks gradually lessen in severity and frequency and usually disappear after

about 18 months. Meanwhile, medication may be prescribed for the acute dizziness.

WAX IN THE EAR

SYMPTOMS

May include: Itching. Pain. Temporary conductive hearing loss.

WHAT TO DO

- **Consult your physician.**
- Home use of wax solvents is not recommended as they may cause allergic reactions and maceration of the skin of the ear canal. Home syringing may be hazardous if infection is present or there is a perforation of the eardrum. Usually, the physician can remove wax readily with little discomfort, using an instrument to roll it out.

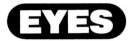

ARCUS SENILIS

SYMPTOMS

Opaque lines around the edges of the corneas, the transparent front covering of the eyes. Usually appears in people over 50 but can occur occasionally at younger ages. Linked with aging. Involves deposit of fat granules.

WHAT TO DO

- No treatment is needed. Arcus senilis does not affect the eyes or sight.

ASTIGMATISM

SYMPTOMS

Vision difficulty caused by inability to focus the eye properly. A congenital defect, astigmatism results from unequal curvature of different areas of the cornea, the transparent front covering of the eye.

WHAT TO DO

- **Consult an eye specialist (ophthalmologist) for suitable eyeglasses.**

BLEPHARITIS

SYMPTOMS

Sensation of a foreign body in the eye. Itching, burning and redness of the eyelid margins. Lid swelling. Loss of lashes. Tearing. Sensitivity to light. An inflammation of the eyelid margins that may result from bacterial infection (usually staph) or allergy.

WHAT TO DO

- **Consult your physician.**
- Treatment may include warm compresses, antibiotic ointment, medicated drops.

CATARACT

SYMPTOMS

Gradual, progressive blurring and dimming of vision. Need for brighter light for reading. Frequent changes of eyeglasses. Sometimes: Double vision. Clouding of the lens of the eye. May result from injury to the eye or from heat or radiation, but mostly occurs with aging.

WHAT TO DO

- **Consult an eye specialist (ophthalmologist).**
- Surgical removal of the clouded lens may be recommended, along with special eyeglasses or contact lens. Sight is restored virtually to normal.

CHOROIDITIS

SYMPTOMS

Blurred vision. The size or shape of objects is distorted. Sometimes: Eye pain. Tearing. An inflammation of the choroid, the middle vascular (blood vessel) coat of the eye, and frequently of the retina as well. The cause is often unknown.

WHAT TO DO

- **Consult an eye specialist (ophthalmologist).**
- Treatment includes medication to suppress inflammation until the cause disappears by itself or can be eliminated, if the problem lies with amebiasis or other treatable problem.

COLOR BLINDNESS

SYMPTOMS

Most commonly: Inability to distinguish between red and green. In rare cases: All colors may appear black and white. Mostly hereditary. Usually transmitted to the male through the mother, who carries the trait from her father though she is not herself affected. Occasionally may result from drugs, injuries or diseases.

WHAT TO DO

- No treatment is available except possibly in those cases where color blindness develops as a result of drugs, injuries or diseases.

CONJUNCTIVITIS ("Pinkeye")

SYMPTOMS

Tearing. Watery discharge later becoming laden with mucus or pus and often sealing the lid margins overnight. Eyelids redden, itch and burn. Sensitivity to light. Inflammation of the conjunctiva, the thin membrane that covers the eyeball and lines the eyelids. Caused by viruses, bacteria or allergy (to pollens, dusts, animal danders, other airborne substances, hair dye, nail polish, face powder). A chronic form, with similar but less severe symptoms, may produce exacerbations and remissions over months and years.

WHAT TO DO

- **Consult your physician.**
- Treatment depends on the suspected cause. Antibiotics or other medication may be prescribed. If caused by an allergy, the suspected substance should be avoided if possible.

CORNEAL ULCER

SYMPTOMS

Eye pain. Sensitivity to light. Tearing. Eye muscle spasm. Ulceration of the cornea, the transparent front covering of the eye. May result from bacteria invading after an injury to the cornea or from spread of infection from other areas.

WHAT TO DO

- **Consult an eye specialist (ophthalmologist).**
- Treatment may include antibiotics applied to the eye and administered by mouth, hot compresses, local anesthetics, patching, cauterization of the base of the ulcer.

DACRYOCYSTITIS

SYMPTOMS

Pain, redness and swelling about the tear sac of the eye. Tearing with pus discharge. Conjunctivitis, redness and swelling of the eyelid margins. Inflammation of the tear sac of the eye. Caused by obstruction of the tear canal (nasolacrimal duct) leading into the nose or by nose injury, deviated septum, nasal polyps or other nasal problems.

WHAT TO DO

- **Consult an eye specialist (ophthalmologist).**
- Treatment may include hot compresses and antibiotics. If abscess has formed, incision and drainage may be required.

DARK GLASSES ABUSE

SYMPTOMS

May produce increased sensitivity to light.

WHAT TO DO

- Unless your physician advises it, avoid constant use of dark glasses. They do cut down glare and, in some cases, have value for eye disorders that produce photophobia, an increased sensitivity to bright lights. But constant wear usually is unnecessary and may be deleterious.

DETACHED RETINA

SYMPTOMS

Light flashes. Sensation of a curtain being drawn across the eye. Detachment of the retina at the back of eye may be caused by accidents and some eye diseases. It is more frequent in people with severe myopia (nearsightedness). The detachment is partial at first but may become complete if not treated promptly.

WHAT TO DO

- **Consult an eye specialist (ophthalmologist) immediately.**
- Early treatment is usually effective. In some cases, reattachment is possible with the use of a laser beam technique.

EXOPHTHALMOS

SYMPTOMS

Eyeball protrusion. Commonly due to excessive thyroid functioning (hyperthyroidism). Other possible causes include clotting in a blood vessel in the eye socket, inflammation, edema (fluid accumulation), tumor, injury.

WHAT TO DO

- **Consult your physician.**
- Treatment depends upon cause. Exophthalmos caused by hyperthyroidism can be effectively controlled. If a tumor is present, surgery may be necessary. Medication may be prescribed to control edema.

EYE DISORDERS FROM DRUGS

SYMPTOMS

Vary. For example: Lens clouding (cataract) may

sometimes result from prednisone or other corticosteroids. Glaucoma may be a side effect of corticosteroids or some drugs used to control high blood pressure. Vision blurring may result from some drugs used for allergies, some tranquilizers, some anti-inflammatory agents. Double vision may occur with some antihistamine drugs for allergies. Other drugs may also produce eye disturbances. These side effects are rare, affecting only a few people.

WHAT TO DO

- **Consult your physician immediately** if you notice a vision or other disturbance developing within days or weeks after starting a drug. He can determine whether the disturbance is caused by a drug and whether a change of dosage or substitution of another drug could avoid the side effects and work just as well for the original problem.

EYE DISORDERS FROM TOBACCO, ALCOHOL (Toxic amblyopia)

SYMPTOMS

Reduced visual acuity, usually in both eyes. A toxic or poisonous reaction in part of the optic nerve. Caused by excessive use of alcohol or tobacco. Sometimes results from chemicals such as lead.

WHAT TO DO

- **Consult an eye specialist (ophthalmologist) immediately.**
- If the diagnosis is toxic amblyopia, vision may improve if the cause is promptly removed.

FARSIGHTEDNESS (Hyperopia)

SYMPTOMS

Blurring of vision at near distances, such as are used for reading and writing, but clear vision at greater distances. The eyeball axis is too short, or the refractive power of the eye is too weak.

WHAT TO DO

- **Consult an eye specialist (ophthalmologist).**
- Can be corrected with properly prescribed eyeglasses.

FLOATERS (Spots)

SYMPTOMS

Spots are seen before one or both eyes. Usually due to debris from the gelatinous substance (vitreous humor) that fills much of the eyeball. More common in highly nearsighted and older people. Tend to become less noticeable with time.

WHAT TO DO

- **Consult an eye specialist (ophthalmologist)** to make certain the spots are innocent floaters. Any disturbance of vision should be investigated.

GLAUCOMA

SYMPTOMS

Symptoms of CHRONIC glaucoma, the most common form: Slowly progressive loss of side vision. When left uncontrolled, later loss of central vision and, ultimately, blindness. Should be suspected in anyone, especially someone over 40, who needs frequent lens changes, suffers mild headaches or vague visual disturbances, sees halos around electric lights or finds it difficult to adjust to the dark. Symptoms of ACUTE glaucoma: May begin with fleeting episodes of reduced visual acuity, seeing colored halos around lights, eye pain, head pain. Episodes may recur at intervals and be followed by a sudden acute attack, with rapid loss of sight, severe throbbing eye pain, nausea and vomiting. Glaucoma is characterized by increased pressure within the eye which can damage the retina and optic nerve. It accounts for almost half of all cases of adult blindness.

WHAT TO DO

- **Consult an eye specialist (ophthalmologist) immediately.** Prompt treatment is essential for acute glaucoma.
- Early diagnosis often allows effective treatment with drugs that reduce intraocular pressure. In some advanced cases, surgery may be recommended to improve drainage of pressure-increasing fluid.
- Early detection is aided by regular medical checkups which include a simple test to measure intraocular pressure.

IRITIS

SYMPTOMS

Severe eye pain which may radiate to the forehead. Vision blurring. Tenderness of the eyeball. Reddened eye. Contracted pupil. An inflammation of the iris, the colored portion of the eye with the pupil in its center. May be associated with tonsillitis, other infection or an injury, but the cause seldom can be identified.

WHAT TO DO

- **Consult an eye specialist (ophthalmologist).**
- Treatment may include dilation of the pupil with medicated drops and other medication to reduce inflammation.

KERATITIS

SYMPTOMS

**May include several of the following: Sensation of a

foreign body in the eye. Tearing. Eye pain. Diminished vision. Sensitivity to light. Inflammation of the cornea, the transparent front covering of the eye. May be caused by bacteria or viruses (including the virus responsible for cold sores and fever blisters).

WHAT TO DO
- **Consult an eye specialist (ophthalmologist).**
- Treatment depends upon the cause. Antibiotics or other drugs may be prescribed.

NEARSIGHTEDNESS (Myopia)

SYMPTOMS

Good near vision but blurring of distant objects. Caused by the inherited shape of the eyeball, which has too long an axis, or too strong a refractive power.

WHAT TO DO
- **Consult an eye specialist (ophthalmologist).**
- Can be corrected with properly prescribed eyeglasses.

OPTIC NEURITIS

SYMPTOMS

Vision disturbance, usually in one eye, ranging from small contraction of the visual field to blindness. An inflammation of the optic nerve. May follow a viral illness or occur with multiple sclerosis, meningitis or syphilis. It can also develop after a beesting or exposure to some chemicals such as lead and wood alcohol. In people over 60, it may result from temporal arteritis.

WHAT TO DO
- **Consult an eye specialist (ophthalmologist).**
- Medication administered by mouth or injected behind the eyeball may be prescribed.

PRESBYOPIA

SYMPTOMS

Difficulty with near vision develops with age. Results from a change in the mechanism which adjusts the focus of the eye for objects at different distances.

WHAT TO DO
- **Consult an eye specialist (ophthalmologist).**
- Can be corrected with properly prescribed eyeglasses.

PTERYGIUM

SYMPTOMS

A winglike patch of thickened conjunctiva membrane grows over part of the cornea, the transparent front covering of the eye. May or may not interfere with sight.

WHAT TO DO
- Not a serious condition. But if the growth interferes with sight, consult an eye specialist (ophthalmologist). Surgical removal may be recommended.

RETINITIS

SYMPTOMS

Reduced visual acuity. Eye discomfort. The size or shape of objects is distorted. An inflammation of the retina in one or both eyes. May be caused by injury, smoking, excessive alcohol use, choroiditis, iritis.

WHAT TO DO
- **Consult an eye specialist (ophthalmologist).**
- Treatment may include elimination of the cause and prescribed medication.

RETINITIS PIGMENTOSA

SYMPTOMS

Narrowing of side vision, producing "tunnel" vision effect. Central vision also frequently reduced by middle age. Defective night vision. An inherited disease causing progressive degeneration of the retina.

WHAT TO DO
- **Consult an eye specialist (ophthalmologist).** Although no treatment is effective at the present time, new experimental therapies may become available.

RETINOPATHIES

SYMPTOMS

May include: Vision blurring. Blood spots in the eyes. Bloodshot appearance. Noninflammatory disease of the retina. May develop from severe high blood pressure, arterio-atherosclerosis, diabetes.

WHAT TO DO
- **Consult your physician.**
- Effective treatment involves treating the underlying disease.
- For an advanced case in which retinal blood vessels may hemorrhage, causing blood spots and vision blurring, treatment with a laser beam may be used to coagulate the vessels.

STRABISMUS ("Cross-eye")

SYMPTOMS

Deviation of an eye. Usually results from unequal eye

muscle tone. Occasionally may stem either in childhood or adulthood from an eye disease or nervous system disease. If not corrected, strabismus may impair vision since, to avoid seeing double, the person may use one eye less or not at all, causing the vision in that eye to deteriorate.

WHAT TO DO
- **Consult an eye specialist (ophthalmologist).**
- Treatment may include corrective glasses or contact lenses, eye exercises, patching the normal eye to encourage use of the other, surgery to restore muscle balance.

STY

SYMPTOMS

Pain, redness and tenderness in the eyelid, followed by the appearance of a small, round, tender pimple-like area. Other symptoms may include: Tearing. Sensitivity to light. Sensation of a foreign body in the eye. An infection of one of the sebaceous glands of the eyelid.

WHAT TO DO
- After the sty has "pointed," producing a small yellowish spot in its center, it may soon rupture, releasing the pus and relieving the pain.
- Pointing can be speeded with hot compresses applied for 10 minutes 3 or 4 times a day.
- In the early stages, pus formation can be stopped with an antibiotic ointment prescribed by a physician.

TEMPORAL ARTERITIS

SYMPTOMS

Headache. Pain and tenderness in the artery running along the temple. A serious possible complication: Sudden blindness in one or both eyes. An inflammation of the temporal artery.

WHAT TO DO
- **Consult your physician immediately.**
- High initial doses of prescribed medication are given to control symptoms and prevent possible blindness. The dosage is gradually reduced.

TRACHOMA

SYMPTOMS

Reddened eyes. The lids swell and stick together, and later become pocked and scarred. The cornea, the transparent front covering of the eye, may become ulcerated. As the disease progresses, vision loss may occur. Caused by an organism, Chlamydia trachomatis. The disease is common in some areas of the Mediterranean and Far East, occurs sporadically among American Indians and in some areas of the southern U.S. Transmitted by direct contact or by handling contaminated towels and other articles. It is most contagious in the early stages.

WHAT TO DO
- **Consult your physician.**
- An antibiotic eye ointment may be prescribed. Treatment is effective.

XANTHELASMA

SYMPTOMS

Soft yellow fat spots on the eyelids. Occurs usually in older people with a genetic disorder of fat metabolism (Type II Hyperlipoproteinemia) which leads to high blood levels of cholesterol and fat deposits on the eyelids.

WHAT TO DO
- **Consult your physician.**
- Diet and, if necessary, drugs to lower cholesterol levels may be prescribed. Consulting a nutritionist can be helpful.
- In some cases, surgical removal of the eyelid spots may be recommended.

HERNIAS

FEMORAL HERNIA

SYMPTOMS

A small or large lump in the thigh, about an inch below the groin (the abdominal wall near where the thigh joins the trunk). More common in women than men. The hernia — a weakening of tissue that may be caused by lifting, coughing or straining at stool — allows a loop of intestine to push out. On lying down, the loop may fall back into the abdomen, but it pushes out again on rising. There is danger that the hernia may become strangulated if the loop becomes caught and constricted in the bulge, with a risk of gangrene.

WHAT TO DO
- **Consult your physician.**
- Temporary treatment may involve wearing a truss. In most cases, surgery provides a cure.

HIATUS HERNIA

In most cases: None. In some cases: Heartburn. Discomfort under the breastbone, sometimes radiating to the left shoulder and arm, occurring soon after meals when lying or bending down. May also include: Vomiting blood. Stools darkened with blood. A protrusion of a small part of the stomach above the diaphragm through a weakened, enlarged diaphragm opening.

•**Consult your physician** to make certain of diagnosis.
•Treatment may consist of relatively simple measures: eating more frequent smaller meals, sleeping with the head of the bed raised on 6- to 8-inch blocks; weight reduction if overweight; avoiding excessive lifting, bending and lying down soon after meals; using antacids. These measures are often effective. If they fail, surgery to repair the opening may be considered.

INGUINAL HERNIA

A small or large lump in the groin (the abdominal wall near where the thigh joins the trunk). The most common type of hernia, it is much more frequent in men than women. The hernia — a weakening of tissue that may be caused by lifting, coughing or straining at stool — allows a loop of intestine to push out, sometimes extending into the scrotum. On lying down, the lump may fall back into the abdomen, but it pushes out again on rising. There is danger that the hernia may become strangulated if the loop becomes caught and constricted in the bulge, with a risk of gangrene.

•**Consult your physician.**
•Temporary treatment may involve wearing a truss. In most cases, surgery provides a cure.

UMBILICAL HERNIA

Protrusion of the navel, most often in an infant, sometimes in a woman after pregnancy. As weak muscles pull away, the abdominal membrane protrudes under the skin and may make the navel look inflated.

•**Consult your physician.**
•Many small umbilical hernias tend to disappear gradually and may need no treatment other than use of adhesive tape or other support. If the hernia persists or has become large enough to admit an adult little finger, surgical repair may be advised when the infant is about a year old. In some cases, surgical repair may also be advisable for an adult.

INFECTIOUS DISEASES: BACTERIAL

ANTHRAX

Red-brown elevation of the skin which grows in size, reddens and blisters. Other symptoms may include: Swelling of nearby lymph nodes. Fever. Muscle aches. Headache. Nausea. Vomiting. Symptoms of a less common form of anthrax that may affect the lungs: Lung congestion. Breathing difficulty. Bluish color. An infectious disease of cattle, horses, mules, sheep and goats. It is only rarely transmitted to humans via contact with an infected animal or animal by-products such as skins.

•**Consult your physician.**
•Antibiotics and other medication may be prescribed. Treatment is usually effective.

BACILLARY DYSENTERY (Shigellosis)

IN CHILDREN: Sudden fever, drowsiness or irritability. Abnormal pain. Straining at stool. Followed within 72 hours by: Diarrhea, with 20 or more stools daily containing blood, pus, mucus. IN MOST ADULTS: No fever. Diarrhea without blood. Little straining at stool. IN SOME ADULTS: Griping abdominal pain relieved by bowel movement. Pain episodes increase in frequency. Diarrhea becomes severe. Stools contain mucus, pus and often blood. An acute bowel infection from Shigella bacteria. Transmitted by food or drink contaminated by the disease carrier.

•**Consult your physician.**

- Antibiotics may be prescribed. A vital part of the treatment is replacement of fluids, sometimes by vein.

BLOOD POISONING
(Bacteremia, septicemia)

SYMPTOMS

Fever, sometimes intermittent, with chills at the onset and wide variations over the day. Skin eruptions with black or blue marks from bleeding into the skin. Caused by bacteria in the circulating blood. May occur with pneumonia, many other infections, tooth extraction, tonsillectomy and other surgery. Sometimes results from minor scratches or cuts.

WHAT TO DO

- **Consult your physician.**
- Hospitalization is usually needed, with intensive administration of antibiotics by injection. Supportive measures include adequate nutrition and fluid intake.

BOTULISM

SYMPTOMS

Blurred sight. Double vision. Drooping of the upper eyelids. Swallowing difficulty. Speaking difficulty. Muscle weakness. Sometimes: Vomiting. Diarrhea. Acute intoxication affecting the nerves and muscles from food contaminated by toxin produced by the organism Clostridium botulinum. The cause is almost always improperly preserved food, mostly home-canned.

WHAT TO DO

- **Consult your physician immediately.** Botulism can be deadly. Requires vigorous treatment.
- Hospitalization is needed. Treatment may include antiserum, intravenous feeding, sedation, oxygen administration, use of respirator. Survivors recover slowly but usually with no permanent aftereffects.

BRUCELLOSIS (Undulant fever)

SYMPTOMS

May begin suddenly with: Chills. Fever. Severe headache. Occasional diarrhea. Can also begin with: Mild malaise. Muscular pain. Headache. Back pain. Rise in evening temperature. Later: Temperature may rise to 104° or 105°F./40° or 40.5°C. in the evening, then fall to near-normal in the morning with profuse sweating. Intermittent fever may persist for 1 to 5 weeks, disappear (along with all the other symptoms), then return repeatedly. An infection transmitted from pigs, goats and cattle, especially through infected milk or carcass. Most frequent among farmers and others working with animals.

WHAT TO DO

- **Consult your physician.**
- Antibiotics and other medication may be prescribed.

CHOLERA

SYMPTOMS

Abrupt, almost constant diarrhea. Great thirst. Reduced urination. Muscle cramps. Weakness. Skin wrinkling. Eye swelling. Sometimes: Bluish color. Stupor. An acute infection by bacterium, Vibrio cholerae, transmitted through contaminated food or water. Rare in the U.S. Occurs mostly in the tropics and India.

WHAT TO DO

- **Consult your physician.**
- Antibiotics may be prescribed. Fluids — by vein as well as mouth — are essential.

GAS GANGRENE

SYMPTOMS

Occur after severe penetrating or crushing injury, usually in an extremity: the wound site becomes very painful. Gas bubbles arise from oozing fluid. Nearby skin may become darkened or black. In severe cases: Delirum. Prostration. Coma. Caused by Clostridium perfringens bacteria.

WHAT TO DO

- **Consult your physician immediately.** Treatment without delay is urgent.
- Treatment may include removal of foreign material and dead tissue from the wound, antibiotics, antitoxin. In some cases, hyperbaric oxygen (treatment in a high pressure chamber) may be used.

LEPROSY (Hansen's disease)

SYMPTOMS

Pink or brown patches on the skin. Loss of sensation. Appearance of small solid swellings (nodules). Fever. Body hair loss. Open sores may appear. Caused by a bacillus, Mycobacterium leprae. Believed transmitted by discharge from the sores of persons already affected with active leprosy, it is in fact one of the least contagious diseases, contracted by fewer than 1 in 20 of those exposed to it. Mostly found in tropical and subtropical areas of Africa, Asia, Latin America. Less than 3,000 known U.S. cases, most of which originated outside the U.S.

WHAT TO DO

- **Consult your physician.**

- Treatment usually is with a drug, dapsone, sometimes combined with an antibiotic.

PLAGUE

SYMPTOMS

Sudden chills. Fever of 103° to 106°F./39.4° to 41.1°C. Painful lymph node swelling, usually in the groin. Other symptoms may include: Vomiting. Thirst. Generalized pain. Headache. Delirium. After the third day, black spots appear. Long called "black plague" because of the spots, bubonic plague is caused by the bacterium Pasteurella pestis transmitted by the fleas on rats and other rodents. **PNEUMONIC PLAGUE, another form, produces: Coughing. Sputum with flecks of blood. Pneumonia.** Both forms are rare.

WHAT TO DO

- **Consult your physician.**
- Treatment with antibiotics is effective in more than 95 percent of the cases.

PSITTACOSIS (Parrot fever)

SYMPTOMS

Fever. Chills. Malaise. Appetite loss. Coughing (dry at first, then producing pus-laden sputum). A form of pneumonia caused by the bacterium Chlamydia psittaci found mostly in parrots, parakeets and lovebirds, less often in poultry, pigeons and canaries. Picked up by humans through inhaling dust from feathers or contact with excreta of infected birds.

WHAT TO DO

- **Consult your physician.**
- Treatment with antibiotics is usually very effective. Other measures include strict bed rest, oxygen if needed, medication for the cough.

RELAPSING FEVER

SYMPTOMS

Sudden chills. High fever. Headache. Vomiting. Muscle pain. Joint pain. Other symptoms may include: Delirium. Reddish rash on the trunk and extremities, followed by rose-colored spots. Jaundice (skin yellowing). Symptoms may disappear after several days or a week or more, then recur at 1- to 2-week intervals. Caused by spirochete bacteria transmitted by ticks and lice. In the U.S., occurs mainly in the western states.

WHAT TO DO

- **Consult your physician.**
- Treatment with antibiotics is effective. Medication may be prescribed for headache and vomiting.

TETANUS (Lockjaw)

SYMPTOMS

May begin with: Jaw stiffness. Swallowing difficulty. Stiff neck, arms or legs. Restlessness. Irritability. Headache. Fever. Sore throat. Chilliness. Sometimes: Convulsions. Later symptoms: Jaw opening becomes difficult. Spasm of the facial muscles produces a fixed smile and eyebrow elevation. An infection caused by bacteria in the soil and dust entering the body through a skin break, especially a puncture wound (nail, splinter, insect bite).

WHAT TO DO

- **Consult your physician immediately.**
- Intensive treatment and almost constant nursing care are required. Treatment usually includes use of antitoxin, medication to control muscle spasm, antibiotics.
- Can and should be prevented by immunization.

TRAVELER'S DIARRHEA

SYMPTOMS

Diarrhea. May be accompanied by: Nausea. Vomiting. Stomach and intestinal sounds. Abdominal cramps. Probably caused by E. coli bacteria. May be transmitted to travelers in less well-developed countries through drinking water, water used for brushing teeth, ice, uncooked food, fruit and vegetables that cannot be peeled.

WHAT TO DO

- Recent medical studies indicate an old patent remedy, Pepto-Bismol, often markedly reduces symptoms within 24 hours when an ounce is taken every half hour for 4 hours.
- **Consult a physician** if the diarrhea persists for several days.

TULAREMIA (Rabbit fever)

SYMPTOMS

Sudden chills. Fever of 103° to 104°F./39.4° to 40°C. Headache. Nausea. Vomiting. Severe prostration. Followed by: Great weakness. Recurring chills and sweats. 24 to 48 hours later, a small sore develops at the site of the infection (finger, eye, arm or the roof of the mouth). At any stage of the disease a generalized red rash may appear. Acute infection by a bacterium, Francisella tularensis, found in wild rabbits and rodents. Most often affected: hunters, butchers, farmers, fur-handlers, laboratory personnel.

WHAT TO DO

- **Consult your physician.**
- Treatment usually includes antibiotics, medication for

intense headache, warm salt-water compresses, and dark glasses when the eyes are affected.

TYPHOID FEVER

SYMPTOMS

Begin gradually with: Chilly sensations. Appetite loss. Headache. Nosebleed. Backache. Constipation. Abdominal pain becomes the most pronounced symptom. If untreated, pneumonia may develop. In a minority of cases: Crops of rose-colored spots on the abdomen and chest. Diarrhea. Infection by S. typhi bacteria transmitted by the stool or urine of persons already affected with the disease and by contaminated water, milk and food.

WHAT TO DO

- **Consult your physician.**
- Treatment usually includes antibiotics, skilled nursing care, fluid replacement.

INFECTIOUS DISEASES: FUNGAL

COCCIDIOIDOMYCOSIS
(Valley fever, San Joaquin fever)

SYMPTOMS

Symptoms of the PRIMARY form, which is benign: Most commonly: Fever. Coughing. Chest pain. May also include: Sore throat. Spitting of blood. Sometimes there are no symptoms. **Symptoms of the PROGRESSIVE form, which infrequently develops from the primary and is chronic and spreading, may include: Low-grade fever. Appetite loss. Weight loss. Strength loss. Breathing difficulty. Bluish color. Sometimes: Bloody sputum.** Caused by the fungus Coccidioides immitis. Acquired by inhaling fungus spore-laden dust. Endemic in the southwestern U.S. Most often affects men aged 25 to 55.

WHAT TO DO

- **Consult your physician.**
- Treatment usually is not needed for the primary disease. But the progressive type can be fatal. Treatment is with an antifungal agent, amphotericin B, which is the only effective drug.

HISTOPLASMOSIS

SYMPTOMS

The PRIMARY ACUTE form produces: Fever. Coughing. Malaise. In a small number of cases, a **PROGRESSIVE DISSEMINATED form, involving spread of infection from the lungs, produces: Liver, spleen and lymph node enlargement. Sometimes: Mouth or gastrointestinal ulceration.** A third form that is **CHRONIC in the lungs produces: Coughing. Increasing breathing difficulty.** Caused by a fungus, Histoplasma capsulatum, inhaled in dust. Occurs all over the U.S., with highest incidence in the Ohio and Mississippi River valleys.

WHAT TO DO

- **Consult your physician.**
- The primary acute form rarely needs treatment. For other forms, an antifungal drug may be prescribed. Treatment often is effective.

INFECTIOUS DISEASES: RICKETTSIAL

ROCKY MOUNTAIN SPOTTED FEVER

SYMPTOMS

Begin with: Abrupt severe headache. Chills. Muscle pains. Prostration. Within 48 hours: Fever of 103° to 104°/39° to 40° C. Followed about fourth day by: Pink, later dark rash starting on the wrists, ankles, palms, soles and forearms, then extending to the neck, face, underarms, buttocks and trunk. Other symptoms may include: Restlessness. Insomnia. Delirium. Caused by tick-borne microscopic parasites called rickettsiae. Once thought confined to the western states of the U.S., the disease actually occurs in many areas, expecially on the Atlantic seaborad.

WHAT TO DO

- **Consult your physician immediately.** Early treatment can avoid complications such as pneumonia and brain and heart damage.
- Treatment with prescribed medication is effective.

TYPHUS

SYMPTOMS

Begin with: Fever rising to about 104°F./40°C. Headache. After 4 to 7 days: Pink spots develop on the upper trunk and rapidly spread to much of the body. Bleeding under the skin. Transmitted by the human body louse and rat fleas.

WHAT TO DO

- **Consult your physician.**
- Treatment with prescribed medication is effective.

INFECTIOUS DISEASES: VIRAL

ACUTE VIRAL HEPATITIS (Infectious and serum hepatitis)

SYMPTOMS

Begin with: Appetite loss. Nausea. Vomiting. Fever. Distaste for cigarettes. Hives. Joint pains. After 3 to 10 days other symptoms may include: Dark urine. Jaundice (yellowed skin). Enlarged, tender liver. Inflamed liver. Enlarged spleen. Two major types of viruses, A and B, are involved; there may also be others. Virus A is spread person-to-person through fecally contaminated water and food. Virus B is transmitted through transfusion of contaminated blood or blood products and through contaminated hypodermic needles. Some medications — such as INH used for tuberculosis, some antidepressants, methyldopa for high blood pressure — may cause hepatitis indistinguishable from the viral form in people overly sensitive to those agents.

WHAT TO DO

- **Consult your physician.**
- In most cases, acute hepatitis clears on its own after 6 to 12 weeks. No special treatment may be needed.

DENGUE (Breakbone fever, dandy fever)

SYMPTOMS

Abrupt chills or chilly sensations. Headache. Pain on moving the eyes. Low back pain. Leg and joint aches. Fever to 104°F./40°C. Prostration. Rash of pale pink spots. Common in the tropics and subtropics. Transmitted by mosquitoes.

WHAT TO DO

- **Consult your physician.**
- Treatment includes bed rest and prescribed medication. Convalescence lasts several weeks.

FLU (Influenza, grippe)

SYMPTOMS

Sudden chilliness. Fever to 102° or 103°F./38.9° or 39.4°C. Aches and pains, especially in the back and legs. Headache. Sore throat. Nonproductive coughing which becomes productive. Often: Sensitivity to light. Acute symptoms subside in 2 to 3 days, but weakness, fatigue and sweating may persist several days longer, in some cases for weeks.

WHAT TO DO

- Bed or other rest is advisable until 24 to 48 hours after the temperature becomes normal. Warm salt water gargles and steam inhalation are helpful. Appropriate medication may relieve the symptoms of fever, cough and nasal obstruction.
- **Consult your physician** if fever, sore throat or coughing persist more than 3 or 4 days, to avoid possible complications such as pneumonia.
- Protection is offered by vaccines.

INFECTIOUS MONONUCLEOSIS (Glandular fever)

SYMPTOMS

Begin with: Malaise. Fatigue. Headache. Chilliness. Followed by: High fever. Sore throat. Generalized lymph node swelling. Other symptoms may include: Jaundice (skin yellowing). Chest pains. Breathing difficulty. Coughing. Eyelid swelling. Although not very contagious, transmitted through close contact, mainly by mouth and nose. High school and college students are especially susceptible.

WHAT TO DO

- **Consult your physician to make certain of diagnosis.**
- No specific drug treatment, but the disease is usually benign and gone in 1 to 4 weeks. Some cases may persist up to 2 to 3 months. Bed rest is important. Salt water gargles are helpful. In severe cases, medication may be prescribed.

RABIES

SYMPTOMS

About a month after an animal bite: Fever. Mental depression. Restlessness. Malaise. Followed by: Great excitation. Excessive salivation. Painful larynx and throat muscle spasms. A dread viral disease, rabies is transmitted by the bite of a rabid animal — a dog, bat, skunk, raccoon, fox or cat.

WHAT TO DO

- **Consult your physician immediately.** Untreated rabies can be fatal. Vaccine treatment is often effective. Treatment with older vaccines required many injections and often had serious side effects, but use of a recently introduced new vaccine requires many fewer injections and is much less likely to produce undesirable effects.
- For first aid for an animal bite, see **BITES & STINGS: ANIMAL BITES** in Part One.

SMALLPOX

SYMPTOMS

Begin with: Chills. High fever. Prostration. May be followed by: Headache. Backache. Muscular pains. On the third day: A rash of small red pustules (pimples) starts on the face, then spreads to the arms, wrists, hands, legs and to some extent to the trunk. 1 or 2 days later: Blisters develop and fill with clear fluid. Subsequently: The fluid turns yellowish and pus-like. The blisters dry up, forming crusts on the skin. After 3 or 4 weeks: The crusts fall off, leaving disfiguring pits. Transmitted person-to-person and by contact with contaminated clothing or other items. Smallpox (also called variola) appears to have been completely eradicated from the earth thanks to a World Health Organization vaccination campaign.

WHAT TO DO

• **Consult your physician immediately** in the unlikely event of symptoms that suggest smallpox.
• Treatment may include rest, nourishment, medication to reduce fever and combat itching, antibiotics for secondary infection.

YELLOW FEVER

SYMPTOMS

Begin with: Sudden fever of 102° to 104°F./38.9° to 40°C. Face flushing. Nausea. Vomiting. Constipation. Abdominal distress. Headache. Muscle pains in the legs, back and neck. Prostration. Restlessness. Later symptoms may include: Jaundice (skin yellowing). Vomiting of blood. Transmitted by mosquito bite. Occurs in central Africa and areas of South and Central America.

WHAT TO DO

• **Consult your physician.**
• Treatment includes bed rest, nursing care, fluid replacement and medication for headache, nausea and vomiting. Blood transfusion is sometimes necessary.

LIVER & GALLBLADDER

CHOLANGITIS

SYMPTOMS

Intermittent, colicky right upper abdominal pain. Jaundice (skin yellowing). Fever. Chills. An inflammation of the bile ducts, which are obstructed by stones or a tumor.

WHAT TO DO

• **Consult your physician.**
• Treatment is usually with antibiotics and fluid replacement. Surgery to overcome the obstruction may be recommended.

CHOLECYSTITIS (Acute)

SYMPTOMS

Right upper abdominal pain which may radiate to the back. Often with: Nausea. Vomiting. Flatulence. Mild fever. Inflammation of the gallbladder. Mostly caused by a gallstone blocking the gallbladder outlet or cystic duct, but sometimes by chemical irritation.

WHAT TO DO

• **Consult your physician.**
• Treatment may include bed rest, antibiotics and other medication. Surgery for removal of the gallbladder may be recommended.

CHOLECYSTITIS (Chronic)

SYMPTOMS

Vary. Some cases limited to: Flatulence. Occasional nausea. In other cases: Pain in the stomach and right upper abdomen. Pain may radiate to the back below the right shoulder blade. Usually appears after a meal or awakens the person at night. The symptoms often follow eating fatty foods. Chronic inflammatory reaction of the gallbladder, the most common kind of gallbladder disease. The cause is not clear.

WHAT TO DO

• **Consult your physician.**
• Surgery may be recommended.

CHOLELITHIASIS (Gallstones)

SYMPTOMS

In some cases: None. In others: Upper abdominal discomfort or pain. Belching. Bloating. Food intolerance. Affects about 10 percent of Americans, more women than men. Involves precipitation of cholesterol from bile, forming stones. The cause is not clear, but there may be increased cholesterol formation and decreased bile synthesis.

WHAT TO DO

• **Consult your physician.**

- Slightly more than half the affected persons experience no pain or only one attack of pain. But since the number likely to experience acute cholecystitis (see **ACUTE CHOLECYSTITIS**) is sizeable, treatment may involve removal of the gallbladder. Now under study is a treatment that attempts to dissolve gallstones by administering bile acids and other agents for several months.

CIRRHOSIS OF THE LIVER

SYMPTOMS

Weakness. Appetite loss. Weight loss. Loss of libido. Malaise. In severe cases symptoms may include: Muscular wasting. Breast enlargement (in men). Hair loss. Testicular wasting. Enlargement of the spleen. Abdominal distention from collection of fluid. A chronic disease involving the degeneration of liver cells and the thickening of surrounding tissues. Most cases occur in middle-aged men from chronic alcoholism. Other causes include severe viral hepatitis, malnutrition, congestive heart failure, syphilis and biliary tract obstruction. A serious disease, cirrhosis is a major killer of 45-to-65-year-olds, ranking right behind heart disease, cancer and stroke.

WHAT TO DO

- **Consult your physician.**
- Treatment may include a high protein diet, multivitamins, a total abstinence from alcohol and, in some cases, medication. Consulting a nutritionist can be helpful.

FATTY LIVER

SYMPTOMS

Usually none, other than painless liver enlargement. Accumulation of fats (triglycerides) in the liver. May be caused by alcohol and various chemicals and drugs such as carbon tetrachloride, tetracycline antibiotics, corticosteroids.

WHAT TO DO

- **Consult your physician.**
- Treatment includes a well-balanced diet, avoidance of alcohol or other causative agents, and weight reduction in the obese. Multivitamins, folic acid and dried brewer's yeast may be prescribed. Consulting a nutritionist can be helpful.

GILBERT'S DISEASE

SYMPTOMS

Usually: Intermittent mild jaundice (skin yellowing). A benign congenital defect in the way the liver handles bilirubin, the bile pigment. Affects up to 5 percent of the population, mostly young adults.

WHAT TO DO

- **Consult your physician.**
- Careful diagnosis is important. The disease is often misdiagnosed as hepatitis. No treatment is available; none is needed. The liver structure remains normal. But it is important to make sure that no consequential disorder is present.

METABOLIC & HORMONAL DISORDERS

ACROMEGALY AND GIGANTISM

SYMPTOMS

Abnormally increased bone length and width. Height may be more than 7 feet. Overgrowth of the mandible and protrusion of the jaw. Coarsening of facial features. Joint pains. Thickened skin. Increased sweating. Results from a benign tumor of the pituitary gland at the base of the brain, which leads to oversecretion of growth hormone.

WHAT TO DO

- **Consult your physician.**

ADDISON'S DISEASE
(Adrenal insufficiency)

SYMPTOMS

Weakness. Fatigue. Low blood pressure on standing or changing position, which may lead to fainting or near-fainting. **Appetite loss. Weight loss. Nausea. Vomiting. Diarrhea. Dark pigmentation of the skin over the knees, elbows and knuckles. Decreased cold tolerance.** Involves a decreased production of some adrenal gland hormones. Sometimes due to tumor, infection or other disease of the adrenals, but in most cases the cause is unknown.

WHAT TO DO

- **Consult your physician.**
- Treatment is usually by daily use of adrenal hormones.

CUSHING'S SYNDROME

SYMPTOMS

May include: Rounded "moon" face. Fat accumulations on the trunk and back ("buffalo hump"). Weakness. Muscle wasting. Thin skin. Easy bruis-

ing. High blood pressure. Kidney stones. Bone thinning and easy fractures. Psychiatric disturbances. Menstrual irregularities. An abnormal increase in adrenal gland secretions. May be due to overactivity of the pituitary gland at the base of the brain, which controls adrenal activity. Sometimes caused by a benign tumor of the adrenal glands or excessive use of corticosteroid hormones.

WHAT TO DO
- **Consult your physician.**
- Treatment depends on the cause. It may include surgery and, if necessary, subsequent daily use of adrenal hormones.

DIABETES INSIPIDUS

SYMPTOMS
Excessive urination and thirst, with drinking and elimination of as many as 40 quarts of fluids daily. Caused by a deficiency of vasopressin, a pituitary gland hormone needed by the kidneys for normal reabsorption of water from the urine. May be congenital or result from injury, tumor or infection.

WHAT TO DO
- **Consult your physician.**
- Treatment may be for the cause if it can be determined. Otherwise, effective control can be obtained with medication.

DIABETES MELLITUS

SYMPTOMS
May begin with: Excessive urination. Followed by: Excessive thirst. Hunger. Weight loss. Later symptoms may include: Appetite loss. Nausea. Vomiting. Increased tendency toward vaginal and other infections. Other possible symptoms include: Impotence. Numbness. Tingling sensation. Vision blurring. Involves inadequate production of insulin by the pancreas, or a disturbance in the body's use of insulin. Occurs in some children. Relatively common after age 40, especially in the obese and those with family histories of diabetes.

WHAT TO DO
- **Consult your physician.**
- Diet, exercise and insulin administration may be used to control the disease. Consulting a nutritionist can be helpful. In milder forms appearing in adulthood, diet and exercise may be adequate; if not, oral anti-diabetes drugs may sometimes be used instead of insulin.

GOITER

SYMPTOMS
Enlargement of the thyroid gland causes a swelling in the front part of the neck. May result from iodine deficiency, or from the effect of some drugs such as aminosalicylic acid and sulfa compounds.

WHAT TO DO
- **Consult your physician.**
- Treatment may be with iodized salt, discontinuance of any drug that may be causing the problem, or use of thyroid hormone.

GOUT

SYMPTOMS
Appear suddenly in an otherwise healthy person, almost always a man. A first attack usually produces throbbing, crushing pain in a joint, most often in a big toe, sometimes in an ankle, instep, knee, wrist or elbow. Later attacks may sometimes affect a different joint, or two or more joints simultaneously. In some cases, may cause: Small painless growths (tophi) in the earlobes and other areas. Formation of kidney stones. Affecting half a million or more Americans, gout is a disorder of the metabolism of purines (substances found in many high protein foods). Uric acid accumulates excessively in the blood, and uric acid crystals are deposited in the joints.

WHAT TO DO
- **Consult your physician.**
- For an acute attack, prescribed medication usually produces dramatic response after 12 hours.
- Other medication is effective in preventing attacks.

HYPERLIPIDEMIA

SYMPTOMS
In some cases, none. In other cases, one or more of the following: Pinkish-yellow fat-deposit lumps around the knees, elbows, buttocks, palms, eyelids and leg and hand tendons. Abdominal pain. Liver enlargement. Spleen enlargement. Involves abnormally high levels of cholesterol and fats (triglycerides) in the blood and tissues. Five different types of hyperlipidemia are recognized. The disorder may result from an inborn fault, diabetes, underfunctioning of the thyroid gland (hypothyroidism), kidney disease, alcoholism, diet or other causes. Associated with a higher risk of coronary artery disease, heart attack, stroke and obstruction of blood vessels in the leg.

WHAT TO DO
- **Consult your physician.**
- Treatment will include correction of any correctable underlying disorder if present. Weight reduction is valuable in obesity, often helping to lower abnormal blood levels. Diet may be prescribed. Consulting a

nutritionist can be helpful. In some cases, medication may be prescribed to reduce abnormal levels.

HYPERPARATHYROIDISM

SYMPTOMS

May include: Appetite loss. Nausea. Abdominal pain. Constipation. Excessive urination. Kidney stones. Results from excessive activity of the parathyroid glands. Possible causes: benign tumor, rarely cancer, of the parathyroids; kidney disease; cancer of the lung, kidney or other organ; other gland disturbances.

WHAT TO DO

- **Consult your physician.**
- Treatment is usually by surgery and correction of other underlying problems.

HYPERTHYROIDISM

SYMPTOMS

May include several of the following: Weakness. Heat sensitivity. Sweating. Overactivity. Weight loss despite increased appetite. Restlessness. Tremors. Eye protrusion. Staring. Sometimes: Headache. Nausea. Abdominal pain. Diarrhea. Involves excessive activity of the thyroid gland. The cause is unknown, but the disease often runs in the family.

WHAT TO DO

- **Consult your physician.**
- Treatment may include antithyroid drugs. Surgery may be recommended.

HYPOGLYCEMIA

SYMPTOMS

May include any of the following: Weakness. Faintness. Palpitation. Hunger. Nervousness. Headache. Confusion. Visual disturbances. Inability to concentrate. Bizarre behavior. A condition in which blood sugar level is abnormally low. May result from organic problems such as tumor of the pancreas, liver disorder, pituitary or adrenal gland dysfunction. Also may result from poor nutrition or severe exertion. In many cases, there is no apparent cause.

WHAT TO DO

- **Consult your physician.**
- Treatment depends upon the cause: A tumor of the pancreas must be removed; a pituitary or adrenal dysfunction will be treated with suitable hormones; etc. Where there is no apparent cause, a high protein – low carbohydrate diet in small meals taken at frequent intervals often helps. Consulting a nutritionist can be helpful.

HYPOPITUITARISM

SYMPTOMS

In CHILDREN: Growth retardation. Small size but normal body proportions. In ADULTS, symptoms may include any of the following: Poor appetite. Weight loss. Fatigability. Cold intolerance. Sparse or absent pubic and underarm hair. Infertility. Lack of menstruation. Deficiency of one or more hormones from the pituitary gland at the base of the brain. May result from various types of brain growths, ballooning of a brain artery, hemorrhage or shock after childbirth, tuberculous or fungus infections that may reach the pituitary.

WHAT TO DO

- **Consult your physician.**
- Treatment is directed at the cause whenever possible. May include surgery, prescribed medication for infection. Treatment also may include replacement of lacking hormones, including those of the pituitary or of the thyroid, adrenal or other glands that are deficient from a lack of normal pituitary stimulation.

HYPOTHYROIDISM

SYMPTOMS

In INFANTS AND CHILDREN with cretinism due to a congenitally absent or grossly inadequate thyroid gland, symptoms may include: Thick, dry skin. Enlarged tongue. Thickened lips. Broad face. Flat nose. Puffy hands and feet. Dull intelligence. In ADULTS, symptoms may include: Slow speech. Dry, thickened skin. Puffy hands and face. Sensitivity to cold. Drowsiness. Mental apathy. Constipation. A deficiency of thyroid hormone. In adults it may result from lack of iodine in the diet, deficient pituitary gland secretion of the hormone thyrotropin which activates the thyroid, or from unknown cause.

WHAT TO DO

- **Consult your physician.**
- Effective treatment requires regular use of thyroid hormone to overcome the deficiency.

PHEOCHROMOCYTOMA

SYMPTOMS

Headache. Palpitation. Tremulousness. Pallor. Sweating. High blood pressure. Abdominal pain. Apprehension. This relatively rare condition is caused by an adrenal gland tumor, usually benign, that produces excessive quantities of adrenal hormones.

WHAT TO DO

- **Consult your physician.**
- Treatment may include use of drugs to block the symptoms. Surgery may be recommended.

PRIMARY ALDOSTERONISM

SYMPTOMS

Episodes of weakness, numbness and tingling. Transient paralysis. High blood pressure. Excessive thirst. Excessive urination. Most often caused by a benign tumor of an adrenal gland, occasionally by a malignant tumor, leading to excessive production of a hormone, aldosterone, which causes sodium retention and potassium loss.

WHAT TO DO
- **Consult your physician.**
- Surgery may be recommended.

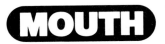

MOUTH

APHTHOUS STOMATITIS
(Canker sores)

SYMPTOMS

Acute painful ulcers of the mucous lining of the mouth, occurring singly or in groups. Often occur 2 or 3 at a time in recurrent attacks, with pain lasting 3 to 4 days and healing, usually without scarring, in 7 to 10 days. In severe attacks: Fever. The cause is unknown. Women are affected more than men, often during menstruation.

WHAT TO DO
- **Consult your physician** for recurrent severe attacks.
- For short-term relief, a topical anesthetic or an antibiotic treatment may be prescribed.

BLACK HAIRY TONGUE

SYMPTOMS

Painless blackening of the tongue. Elongation of the papillae, the thread-like elevations covering the tongue. Often follows an antibiotic treatment that kills many bacteria, allowing an overgrowth of fungi.

WHAT TO DO
- **Consult your physician.**
- An antifungal medication may be prescribed.
- Brushing the tongue may help.

BROKEN OR CHIPPED TOOTH

SYMPTOMS

None immediately except possibly some discomfort from the tongue or cheek rubbing against the tooth. But if the pulp is exposed, infection and abscess formation may follow.

WHAT TO DO
- **Consult your dentist.**

- Prompt treatment can save the pulp and tooth and help avoid infection.

BRUXISM

SYMPTOMS

Grinding of the teeth, usually when asleep. May damage teeth and possibly the gums.

WHAT TO DO
- **Consult your dentist.**
- An appliance called a biteplate used in the mouth during sleep may prevent the grinding.

DENTAL CARIES (Cavities)

SYMPTOMS

Decay-produced cavity which, if untreated, may affect the pulp of the tooth, causing pain and possible swelling of the face. Caused by dissolution of the enamel and dentin of the tooth by acid produced by bacteria in a film called plaque.

WHAT TO DO
- **Consult your dentist.**
- Treatment requires filling the tooth.
- Most cavities can be prevented by eliminating the build up of plaque through proper brushing and flossing.

GANGRENOUS STOMATITIS

SYMPTOMS

Appearance of gray-black tissue on the gums or inside the cheeks or lips. Swollen cheeks, which may become red, then black on the outside. Pain. Fever. A serious gangrene (tissue death). May occur in undernourished, weakened elderly people and children. Sometimes develops in young children with complications from measles or whooping cough.

WHAT TO DO
- **Consult your physician immediately.**
- Antibiotics may be prescribed.

GEOGRAPHIC TONGUE

SYMPTOMS

White or pinkish patches of spots that keep changing from day to day. Usually not painful. May occur in children and young adults, especially those under stress or with allergies or histories of allergies.

WHAT TO DO
- **Consult your physician.**
- No specific treatment, but the physician can give assurance that there is no danger of cancer or serious illness.

GINGIVITIS

SYMPTOMS

Swollen, red, bleeding gums. Inflammation of the gums. Commonly caused by bacteria growing in a film of plaque on the teeth. May also result from tartar (calculus), malocclusion, food impaction. Can be the first indication of vitamin deficiencies, allergy, blood disorders or other systemic disease. Sometimes results from long use of an anticonvulsant drug, phenytoin.

WHAT TO DO
- **Consult your dentist.**
- Tartar must be removed. Malocclusion or other local cause must be corrected. If there is underlying systemic disease, it must be treated. A program of good oral hygiene, involving regular dental visits and proper brushing and flossing at home, should be established.

GLOSSITIS

SYMPTOMS

Vary. In some cases, the tip and edges of the tongue become red. (May indicate pellagra, pernicious anemia, excessive smoking or irritation from a tooth.) In other cases, there are painful ulcers on the tongue. (May indicate viral or other infection.) In still other cases, white patches appear on the tongue. (May indicate fungal infection, mouth breathing or other problems.) An inflammation of the tongue.

WHAT TO DO
- **Consult your physician.**
- Glossitis requires careful study to determine and treat the cause. Treatment may include avoiding alcohol, smoking, spices and hot drinks, and practicing good oral hygiene including care of the teeth.

GLOSSODYNIA

SYMPTOMS

Painful burning tongue with no evidence of inflammation. Often occurs in postmenopausal women. May be psychosomatic but may also be related to anemia, diabetes mellitus or nutritional deficiencies.

WHAT TO DO
- **Consult your physician.**
- Treatment is for cause.

HERPES LABIALIS
(Cold sores, fever blisters)

SYMPTOMS

Itching and burning about the lips, followed by blisters, then crusted sores which may persist for a week or so before healing. Caused by a virus infection which may develop from any disease that produces a fever or from sunburn, food allergy, onset of menstruation.

WHAT TO DO
- Application of 70 percent isopropyl alcohol may reduce the itching and burning before the blisters appear and have a drying effect when the blisters ooze. Petrolatum applied on crusted sores may help.
- **Consult your physician** for frequently recurring outbreaks.

IMPACTED TOOTH

SYMPTOMS

Possible inflammation, pain and swelling of the gum surrounding a tooth, most often a third molar that fails to erupt above the gum line.

WHAT TO DO
- **Consult your dentist.**
- Treatment may include antibiotic treatment as well as dental efforts to help the tooth erupt.

KNOCKED OUT TOOTH

WHAT TO DO
- **Consult your dentist immediately.** If the tooth can be reimplanted within 30 minutes, chances are the interior pulp will survive. Even up to 6 hours, reimplantation may be possible. If there is to be a delay, try putting the tooth in the socket yourself. If that isn't possible, place the tooth in a container of water or wrap it in cloth wetted with water to which a little salt has been added — and hurry to dentist.

LEUKOPLAKIA

SYMPTOMS

White patches in some part of the mouth, most often on the inside of the cheeks, the tongue or the floor of the mouth. More common in men than women. The greatest incidence is between ages 40 and 70. May result from smoking, alcohol, cheek biting, sharp worn-down teeth, ill-fitting dentures, spicy food, vitamin deficiency. Sometimes, precancerous.

WHAT TO DO

- **Consult your dentist.**
- Any dental problems contributing to leukoplakia should be corrected. Tobacco and other irritants should be eliminated. Treatment may include removal or cauterization of small, local patches.

MALOCCLUSION

SYMPTOMS

Imperfect contact between upper and lower teeth. Among the many possible causes: teeth too large for the jaw to accommodate; malformed or missing teeth; delayed eruption of permanent teeth above the gum line; early loss of teeth from decay or gum disease.

WHAT TO DO

- **Consult your dentist.**
- Can be corrected by orthodontic treatment with braces or other measures. Treatment will improve appearance and contribute to health by increasing resistance to decay and gum disease, and improving chewing and digestion.

ORAL LICHEN PLANUS

SYMPTOMS

Bluish-white lesions on the inside of the cheek and tongue margins. May increase in size, become ulcerated, painful. Repeated exacerbations and remissions may occur. Basically, lichen planus is an inflammatory eruption of the skin. The mouth is involved in about half the cases and is often affected before the skin is. (See also **LICHEN PLANUS.**) The cause is unknown.

WHAT TO DO

- **Consult your physician.**

PERIODONTITIS (Pyorrhea)

SYMPTOMS

Deepening of pockets between the gum and teeth lead to debris collecting in the pockets, multiplication of bacteria, pus formation, loss of bone, loosening of teeth. Periodontitis is a progression of untreated gingivitis and results from the same causes; see **GINGIVITIS.**

WHAT TO DO

- **Consult your dentist.**
- Treatment includes correction of any irritating factors in the mouth and instruction in home care. Advanced periodontitis may require surgery and reconstruction of the gum tissues.

PERLECHE

SYMPTOMS

Inflammation and reddening of the corners of the mouth. Sometimes with: Fissuring or ulceration. Painful burning. May result from ill-fitting dentures, smoking, possibly malnutrition.

WHAT TO DO

- **Consult your physician.**
- Treatment includes correction of any apparent cause. In some cases, medicated ointment may be prescribed.

PULPITIS

SYMPTOMS

Sharp, shooting mouth pain. May be intermittent and difficult to localize, possibly seeming to come from the opposite side of the jaw. An inflammation of the dental pulp, the soft white tissue within a tooth. Most frequently caused by a cavity. May sometimes result from an injury or a thermal or chemical irritation.

WHAT TO DO

- **Consult your dentist.**
- In early cases, removing food debris from the cavity and packing it with clove oil, or clove oil mixed with zinc oxide powder may offer relief. In advanced cases, root canal therapy or tooth removal may be required.

RANULA (Mouth cyst)

SYMPTOMS

A cyst or sac on the underside of the tongue (ranula), accompanied by discomfort or, if inflamed, pain. Or a cyst of the small glands in the cheek, lip or palate (mucocele).

WHAT TO DO

- **Consult your physician.**
- The discomfort of a ranula may be relieved by removing the fluid with needle suction. Surgery may be recommended. A mucocele commonly ruptures on its own and heals. In case of recurrence, surgery may be advised.

SCROTAL TONGUE

SYMPTOMS

Deep grooves in the tongue surface. Accompanied by tongue inflammation if food and bacteria become trapped in the grooves. Usually a harmless congenital condition.

WHAT TO DO

- **No treatment is needed unless infection sets in.**
- **In case of infection, consult your physician.** Antibiotics may be prescribed.

STOMATITIS TRAUMATICA

SYMPTOMS

Mouth pain. Excessive salivation. May be caused by cheek biting, breathing through the mouth, jagged teeth, poorly fitted dentures, a nursing bottle with a hard or overlong nipple.

WHAT TO DO

- **Consult your dentist.**
- The underlying cause will have to be corrected.

TEMPOROMANDIBULAR JOINT DISORDER

SYMPTOMS

May include: Face pain. Pain in front of an ear. Limited jaw motion because of pain and spasm. Clicking or grating sounds on chewing. The temporomandibular joint connects the upper and lower jaw on each side of the face. Symptoms develop when the joint is affected by arthritis, malocclusion, grinding of the teeth, poorly fitted dentures or emotional disturbances.

WHAT TO DO

- **Consult your physician.**
- Treatment may include heat applications, medication, soft diet for a short period.
- Consultation with a dentist, and bite adjustment or correction of other dental causes may be needed.

THRUSH

SYMPTOMS

White, slightly raised, milk-curd-like patches usually appear first on the tongue and inside the cheeks and may spread to the gums, palate, tonsils, larynx. The mouth usually seems dry. A fungus (Candida albicans) infection which may follow use of antibiotics which, in decimating bacteria, allow room for fungus overgrowth.

WHAT TO DO

- **Consult your physician.**
- An oral rinse containing an antifungal drug may be prescribed.

TONGUE-TIE

SYMPTOMS

Limited mobility of the tongue. Speech defect. A congenital condition in which the mucous membrane connecting the tongue to the mouth floor extends close to the tongue tip.

WHAT TO DO

- **Consult your physician.**
- Surgery may be recommended.

TOOTH ABRASION

SYMPTOMS

Wearing away of and notching in of tooth substance. May be caused by faulty brushing, pipe smoking, frequent holding of nails, pins, other objects between the teeth.

WHAT TO DO

- **Consult your dentist.**
- Where loss is substantial, filling may be required to help prevent decay. Demonstration of proper brushing technique may be advisable. Any other contributing factor will also have to be corrected.

TOOTH ABSCESS

SYMPTOMS

Gnawing continuous pain, increased by hot or cold foods. If treatment is delayed, may be followed by: Facial swelling. Fever. Usually caused by infection of the pulp due to decay. Sometimes may occur after tooth injury.

WHAT TO DO

- **Consult your dentist.**
- Extraction or root canal therapy is usually required. Medication may be prescribed for pain and high fever. Bed rest and soft diet sometimes are advisable.

TRENCH MOUTH (Vincent's infection)

SYMPTOMS

Painful bleeding gums. Excessive salivation. Bad breath. Ulcers on the gums and inside the cheeks, covered by grayish membrane. A noncontagious bacterial infection. Often, there is a predisposition because of poor oral hygiene, nutritional deficiency, stress, blood disorder, debilitating disease, insufficient rest.

WHAT TO DO
- **Consult your dentist.**
- Treated by gentle removal of disease-produced foreign material and establishment of good oral hygiene. In acute stages, mouth rinsing with warm salt water or 3 percent peroxide solution may be helpful. Medication may be prescribed for pain. Marked improvement often occurs within 24 hours, after which further removal of foreign material can be carried out. Antibiotic treatment is seldom needed.

TUMORS OF THE MOUTH

SYMPTOMS
Growths on the gums, palate, tongue, lip, cheek or the floor of the mouth. Usually are not painful in the early stages.

WHAT TO DO
- **Consult your physician** for any mouth ulcer or sore that does not heal in 2 weeks. Although it may well be benign, it should be regarded as possibly cancerous until proved otherwise. Diagnosis can be made by examination of a small sample under a microscope.
- Can be cured by early treatment.

MUSCULOSKELETAL SYSTEM

ANKYLOSING SPONDYLITIS

SYMPTOMS
May begin with: Episodes of low back pain. Morning back stiffness. Symptoms become progressively worse with time, spreading from lower to middle back and sometimes into the neck area. In severe cases, symptoms may include: Fatigue. Weight loss. Mild anemia. Muscle stiffness. A chronic progressive arthritic disease of the small joints of the spine.

WHAT TO DO
- **Consult your physician.**
- No curative treatment. But medication may be prescribed to relieve symptoms. Posture-maintaining exercises are important. Hot baths or packs before exercises help. A back brace may or may not be necessary. Only rarely is spinal surgery required.

BUNION

SYMPTOMS
Swelling of the bursa or sac of the first joint below the base of the big toe, producing pain. Results from tight shoes.

WHAT TO DO
- A mild case may be relieved by avoiding shoes with high heels and narrow toes. It may be helpful to switch to "bunion last" shoes with a wide forefoot section.
- **Consult your physician for a persistently painful bunion.** Surgery may be recommended.

BURSITIS

SYMPTOMS
Severe pain and limited movement of the affected joint. Inflammation of a bursa, a small fluid-filled sac that enables one part of a joint to move readily over another part or over other structures. The most important bursae are those in the shoulder, elbow, hip and knee. Inflammation develops as a result of injury, infection, excessive use or chilling. **HOUSEMAID'S KNEE** may result from repeated kneeling and bruising. **TENNIS ELBOW,** also known as radiohumeral bursitis, with pain radiating from the elbow to the outer side of the arm and forearm, may result from an activity such as using a screwdriver, as well as playing tennis.

WHAT TO DO
- **Consult your physician.**
- Medication may be prescribed for pain. Rest and splinting are moderately effective.

CONGENITAL HIP DISLOCATION

SYMPTOMS
Not obvious, but the dislocation is often detected when a baby is examined soon after birth or during periodic checkups during the first year. Can involve one or both hips. More common in girls. The cause is unknown.

WHAT TO DO
- **Consult your physician.**

- With early treatment soon after birth, the dislocation can be readily corrected. Treatment becomes more difficult with growth.

DISLOCATION OF SHOULDER

SYMPTOMS

Painful motion. The shoulder looks disjointed. Usually caused by swimming or other vigorous activity, although in some cases it may occur as the result of ordinary movement.

WHAT TO DO

- **Consult your physician.**
- A shoulder should be relocated only by a physician.

FLATFOOT

SYMPTOMS

In some cases: None. In other cases: Pain in the arch that may extend to calf muscles and sometimes to the knee, hip, lower back. Increased by walking or standing. Absence of a normal arch in the sole of the foot.

WHAT TO DO

- Arch supports help while walking. Warm footbaths and rest may reduce discomfort.

FROZEN SHOULDER

SYMPTOMS

Pain deep in the shoulder. Worsens at night. May sometimes extend to the arm, chest or back. Limitation of motion. May result from injury, bursitis, unknown cause. Involves adhesions.

WHAT TO DO

- **Consult your physician.**
- Treatment may include application of heat, prescription of exercises. In severe cases, skilled manipulation by a specialist may be needed to free the adhesions.

GANGLION OF THE WRIST

SYMPTOMS

Painless lump on the back of the wrist. The ganglion is a cyst, a liquid-containing sac.

WHAT TO DO

- Often disappears on its own.
- **In stubborn cases, consult your physician.**

GONOCOCCAL ARTHRITIS

SYMPTOMS

Hot, red, tender joints. Pain on movement. Most often affected: knee, wrist, ankle. May include symptoms of gonorrhea. In a MAN: Painful burning sensation during urination. Whitish discharge. In a WOMAN: Lower abdominal pain with or without burning sensation during urination or whitish vaginal discharge. Caused by gonococcus organisms invading the joints.

WHAT TO DO

- **Consult your physician.**
- Injections of antibiotics may be prescribed.

INGROWN TOENAIL

SYMPTOMS

Toe pain. Redness and swelling if infection develops. Almost always the result of improper toenail trimming or poorly fitting shoes.

WHAT TO DO

- If the ingrowth is only slight, a bit of cotton soaked in caster oil may be inserted under the ingrown nail edge. To protect the nail from pressure, a gauze pad can be applied.
- **If the nail is badly ingrown, consult your physician or podiatrist.** Expert treatment can help prevent infection.
- For prevention, keep the nails short, the sides a little longer than the middle.

JUVENILE RHEUMATOID ARTHRITIS

SYMPTOMS

May begin with: Fever. Rash. Spleen and generalized lymph node enlargement. Followed by: Joint pain or tenderness. Sometimes: Iritis; see IRITIS. Inflammation of the joints. The cause is unknown.

WHAT TO DO

- **Consult your physician.**
- Treratment may include medication, exercises, splints.

LEGG-PERTHES' DISEASE

SYMPTOMS

In a child, usually a boy aged 3 to 9: Limping. Pain in the groin or possibly in the leg, hip or knee. The disease involves impairment of blood flow to the head of the thighbone (femur), which may cause the bone to deteriorate.

- Consult your physician.
- Treatment may require extended bed rest and use of a brace.

LOW BACK PAIN

SYMPTOMS

Sudden severe pain low in the back. Walking difficulty. Standing difficulty. An **ACUTE** pain may result from heavy lifting, a fall, bending over, shoveling, other activity. **CHRONIC** low back pain may be caused by poor posture, obesity, lack of exercise (particularly of the abdominal muscles, so that an added burden is borne by the back muscles). Osteoarthritis of the spine may also be a factor.

WHAT TO DO

- Often, acute low back pain improves after several days of rest on a firm mattress supported by a bed board. Warm moist packs should relieve muscle spasm, an important factor in the pain.
- Consult your physician for chronic low back pain. Treatment may require weight reduction, exercise, posture improvement. A corset may sometimes be useful. If a difference in leg length is a contributing factor, a shoe lift may be helpful.

OSTEOARTHRITIS
(Degenerative joint disease)

SYMPTOMS

Pain in one or a few joints, which increases after exercise. Stiffness after inactivity, usually lasting no more than 15 to 30 minutes. The affected joints may grate or "creak" on movement. They may become enlarged. Especially in women, the small finger joints may become swollen. The most common form of arthritis, involving loss of cartilage in the joints. The cause is unknown. Prevalence is greater in men before age 45, in women after 45.

WHAT TO DO

- Consult your physician.
- Treatment may include weight reduction where necessary; medication to relieve pain and improve mobility, applications of heat. In very severe cases, the joint in the hip, knee or elsewhere can be replaced.

OSTEOMYELITIS

SYMPTOMS

Sudden pain in a bone. Tenderness. Painful movement. Swelling. Fever. An infection of the bone by bacteria. The bacteria may reach the bone through a fracture or other injury, from a nearby infection or through the blood. If the infection becomes chronic, pus may be discharged through an opening over the infected bone, causing flare-ups of pain and destruction of areas of bone.

WHAT TO DO

- Consult your physician immediately.
- Prompt treatment with antibiotics can usually control the infection, minimizing risk of chronic infection. The infected bone is usually immobilized in a cast. If delayed until some bone is destroyed, treatment is more difficult. In chronic osteomyelitis, dead bone will be removed and intensive antibiotic treatment used.

OSTEOPOROSIS

SYMPTOMS

May include: Pain in the vertebrae of the spine, often from the middle back down. Rounding of the shoulders. Loss of height. Tendency for bones to break easily. A loss of bone density, with the bones becoming porous and brittle. Most commonly affects women after menopause but occurs to some extent in both men and women at younger ages. The cause is not understood.

WHAT TO DO

- Consult your physician.
- Treatment may include diet (at least 2 glasses of milk daily), calcium and vitamin D supplements, in some cases sex hormones. Sodium fluoride may sometimes be used. For severe acute back pain, medication, an orthopedic support, heat and massage may be prescribed.

PAGET'S DISEASE (Osteitis deformans)

SYMPTOMS

Bone pain, most commonly in the pelvis, legs, skull, vertebrae, collarbone, arm. Bone thickening, enlargement and deformity. Possible hearing impairment if the temporal bone is affected. A slowly progressive bone disorder of unknown cause, with some tendency to run in families. Occurs mostly after age 40. Affects men more often than women.

WHAT TO DO

- Consult your physician.
- Treatment may include sex hormones, fluoride, medication for pain. Newer treatments are reported to show some promise.

RHEUMATOID ARTHRITIS

SYMPTOMS

May begin with: Fleeting pains in some joints.

Weight loss. Joint stiffness. Fever. In some cases, many joints may be involved from the beginning; in others, involvement may be progressive. Any joints may be affected, but the most common are the small hand joints, feet, wrists, elbows, ankles. Typically affects both sides of the body. Involved joints are tender, with pain that may range from mild to severe. Deformities may develop. A chronic inflammatory disease of the joints, affecting women 2 to 3 times as often as men. Begins at any age but most often after 35. The cause is unknown.

WHAT TO DO

- **Consult your physician immediately.**
- Early treatment is important. Most patients improve with conservative treatment during the first year. With effective early treatment, deformities may be avoided. Medication may be prescribed to relieve inflammation. Exercise helps prevent joint stiffening. Local heat may help relieve spasm and pain. In some cases, surgery may be recommended to remove overgrown, inflamed joint tissue, loosen tendons or ligaments distorting a joint, or replace a severely diseased joint with an artificial joint.

SLIPPED DISC (Ruptured disc, sciatica)

SYMPTOMS

Low back pain. Sometimes: Pain radiating down the thigh and leg to the ankle — sciatica, more severe than the back pain. Cartilage discs between the vertebrae of the spine act like cushions for shock. Rupture of a disc may cause extrusion of the inner material, the nucleus pulposis, causing an inflammatory reaction and back pain. If the material presses the root of the sciatic nerve which extends down the leg, sciatica develops. Disc rupture may be related to injury or to joint degeneration.

WHAT TO DO

- **Consult your physician.**
- Treatment may include bed rest, traction, hot wet applications, medication. Such treatment is usually successful. When it is not, surgery may be recommended.

SPINAL CURVATURE

SYMPTOMS

May take various forms: Round shoulders. A bend in the foreward curve of the lower spine (lordosis, or swayback). Lateral or sideward curvature (scoliosis) with unevenness of the hips or shoulders. The cause usually is unknown, but it may be extended faulty posture, lack of muscle tone from physical inactivity, or rickets. Scoliosis is much more common in girls than boys.

WHAT TO DO

- **Consult your physician immediately.**

- Early treatment is important. The type of treatment depends upon the cause and degree of the problem. Corrective exercises may be effective in some cases; in others, braces, casts or surgery may be recommended.

SPRAINED ANKLE

SYMPTOMS

Swelling. Tenderness. Pain on motion. Sometimes: Skin discoloration. Injury to the soft tissue surrounding the joint, with stretching, sometimes tearing, of ligaments, muscles, tendons, blood vessels.

WHAT TO DO

- **Consult your physician.**
- X-ray may be needed to make certain no bone fracture has occurred.
- Treatment may include rest, elevation of the ankle, cold compresses to help reduce swelling and pain. A walking cast may be needed.

SPRAINED OR STRAINED WRIST

SYMPTOMS

Swelling. Pain. Skin discoloration. SPRAIN involves injury to the soft tissues surrounding a joint, with stretching, sometimes tearing of the ligaments, muscles, tendons, blood vessels. **STRAIN** is a muscle injury, with muscle fibers stretched, sometimes partially torn.

WHAT TO DO

- **Consult your physician.**
- X-ray may be needed to make certain no bone fracture has occurred.
- Treatment may include elastic bandaging of the wrist, ice packs for swelling.

STIFF NECK

SYMPTOMS

Obvious neck stiffness. Mostly a mild disorder from muscle cramp due to an awkward sleeping position, unusual activity, sudden twist of the neck, or chill. Occasionally may be due to arthritis. **In WRYNECK (also called SPASMODIC TORTICOLLIS), the head may be twisted to one side and bent abnormally** due to a spasm or an involuntary contraction of the neck muscles. May be a result of tumor or infection, but the cause usually is unknown.

WHAT TO DO

- Stiff neck can usually be managed well with home measures: hot showers, hot wet packs, massage.
- **If it persists, consult your physician.**
- **For wryneck, consult your physician.**
- Wryneck sometimes may be helped, at least temporari-

ly, by slight pressure on the jaw on the side to which the head is rotated.

TRICK KNEE

SYMPTOMS

Sudden locking or collapse of the knee. May be due to a torn cartilage, some of which may get caught in the knee joint.

WHAT TO DO

- **Consult your physician.**
- Treatment may include manipulation, splinting, removal of bloody fluid by suction with a needle. In some cases, surgery may be recommended.

TUBERCULOSIS OF JOINTS AND BONES

SYMPTOMS

May include: Swelling. Limited motion mainly in the spine or knees, but sometimes in the hip. **Sometimes: Weakness. Stiffness. Limp.** Caused by the organism responsible for lung tuberculosis. Usually results from lung TB. Rare in the U.S.

WHAT TO DO

- **Consult your physician.**
- Treatment is the same as for lung tuberculosis.

WHIPLASH INJURY

SYMPTOMS

Neck pain or stiffness occurring after an injury, usually an automobile accident in which the victim's car is struck from behind and his head is snapped back and forward. Other symptoms may include: Headache. Vision disturbances. May involve muscle spasm, strain or tear of the muscles and ligaments in the neck area.

WHAT TO DO

- **Consult your physician.**
- Treatment may include some or all of the following: heat, medication, traction, use of a cervical collar.

NOSE & THROAT

ADENOID HYPERTROPHY (Enlargement)

SYMPTOMS

May include: Breathing through the mouth. Postnasal discharge. Halitosis. Nasal speech. Coughing. Dull facial expression. Ear pain. Ear pressure. Diminished hearing. Most common in children, enlargement of adenoid tissue in the throat area may obstruct the openings of eustachian tubes leading to the ears. Enlargement may result from infection or allergy, or be without apparent cause.

WHAT TO DO

- **Consult your physician.**
- For persistent symptoms, adenoidectomy — removal of the obstructing tissue — may be recommended.

BENIGN VOCAL CORD GROWTHS

SYMPTOMS

Hoarseness. Breathy voice quality. Caused by polyps or growths on the vocal cords due to voice abuse, allergy, smoking, industrial fumes. The growths are usually benign. The same symptoms may occur as the result of vocal cord nodules due to ongoing voice abuse such as screaming or shouting. (Sometimes called "Singer's," "Teacher's" or "Screamer's Nodules.")

WHAT TO DO

- **Consult your physician.**
- Treatment involves surgical removal of polyps or nodules and correction of voice abuse or other cause to prevent recurrence.

CHRONIC RHINITIS

SYMPTOMS

May include: Obstructed breathing. Nasal discharge. Postnasal drip. Throat tickle. Coated tongue. Dry lips. Headache. Chronic inflammation that may produce thickening of the nasal mucous membrane and enlargement of nasal turbinate structures. May result from repeated upper respiratory infections, chronic sinusitis, polyps, deviated septum, abuse of nose drops.

WHAT TO DO

- **Consult your physician.**
- If possible, any detected cause should be eliminated.

COMMON COLD

SYMPTOMS

Because colds can be produced by different viruses, symptoms may differ. Commonly, they include: Feeling of throat irritation. Sneezing. Runny nose. Feeling of a stuffy head. Slight headache. Eye watering. General aching. Listlessness. Sometimes: Hacking cough. Laryngitis. Fever (especially in a child). Transmitted by droplets through coughing, sneezing and contact with objects on which the droplets have been deposited.

WHAT TO DO

- Rest, steam inhalations and large fluid intake are helpful. Use of vitamin C in large doses — 2 grams or more daily — remains controversial but can be effective.
- **To prevent possible bacterial infection complications, consult your physician if the cold gets worse:** if there are prolonged chills; fever about 103°F./39.4°C.; aches in the chest, ears or face; shortness of breath; persistent hoarseness; coughing up of blood or rust-colored sputum.

DEVIATED SEPTUM

SYMPTOMS

Somewhat difficult breathing. Sometimes: Headache. Postnasal discharge. The septum, a plate of bone and cartilage covered with mucous membrane that divides the nasal cavity, may deviate because of malformation or injury so that one side of the cavity is smaller than the other.

WHAT TO DO

- **Consult your physician.**
- If necessary, surgery may be recommended to relieve obstruction and irritation.

HAY FEVER AND ALLERGIC RHINITIS

SYMPTOMS

Itching nose, roof of mouth, throat, eyes. Eye tearing. Sneezing. Nasal discharge. Sometimes: Headache. Irritability. Wheezing. Coughing. Allergic rhinitis is known as hay fever when it occurs seasonally, as perennial allergic rhinitis when it occurs year-round. It may be caused by pollens, dust, feathers, animal dander.

WHAT TO DO

- **Consult your physician.**
- Medication may be prescribed. Filtered air conditioning may be helpful for hay fever. If possible, avoiding or eliminating causative materials can be valuable for perennial rhinitis.

LARYNGITIS

SYMPTOMS

Hoarseness or loss of voice. Throat tickling and rawness. Repeated efforts to clear the throat. In severe cases, symptoms may include: Fever. Throat pain. Swallowing difficulty. Breathing difficulty. An inflammation of the larynx, or voice box. May result from colds, other respiratory infections, misuse of the voice. Chronic laryngitis, with similar but sometimes less severe symptoms, may result from repeated attacks of acute laryngitis or excessive use of alcohol, smoking, voice abuse, irritating fumes or dusts, chronic inflammation of the nose, tonsils or sinuses.

WHAT TO DO

- **Consult your physician.**
- Treatment may include resting the voice, steam inhalation, warm fluids. Antibiotics may be prescribed if there is a bacterial infection. In chronic laryngitis, the cause should be eliminated if possible.

NASAL POLYPS

SYMPTOMS

May include: Nasal obstruction. Nasal discharge. Sometimes, if the polyps grow large: Headache. Polyps are growths extending out from the mucous membrane. They resemble peeled seedless grapes. May occur in acute and chronic infections or result from allergy.

WHAT TO DO

- **Consult your physician.**
- Treatment may be needed for allergy or infection. If polyps continue to cause trouble, surgical removal may be recommended.

PHARYNGITIS

SYMPTOMS

Sore throat. Pain on swallowing. Fever. Enlarged lymph nodes in the neck area. Inflammation of the pharynx, the 5-inch-long cavity behind the nose, mouth and larynx. May be caused by a common cold, other viral infections, bacterial infections.

WHAT TO DO

- **Consult your physician.**
- Treatment may include rest, warm salt water gargles. Antibiotics may be used if the causative organisms are identified as bacteria.

POSTNASAL DRIP

SYMPTOMS

Repeated efforts to clear the throat. Sometimes:

Coughing. Mostly from mucus secretion (by nasal glands) which may be habitually drawn into the back of the throat instead of allowed to drain through the nose. May also result from allergy, sinus infection, dust or other irritation of the nose.

WHAT TO DO
- Sleeping in a humidified room, or use of a vaporizer at night, may be helpful. So will avoiding drawing mucus into the throat, possibly coupled with increased gentle nose blowing.
- **Consult your physician** if you suspect that allergy or sinusitis might be the cause.

QUINSY (Peritonsillar abscess)

SYMPTOMS

Severe pain on swallowing. Fever. Head held tilted to one side. Sometimes: Marked difficulty in opening the jaw. An abscess between one side of a tonsil and a nearby muscle of the pharynx. Usually caused by strep bacteria.

WHAT TO DO
- **Consult your physician.**
- Treated with antibiotics.
- Because there is a tendency to recurrence, surgical removal of the tonsil may be recommended.

SINUSITIS

SYMPTOMS

May include: Headache. Nasal and postnasal discharge. Toothache. Puffiness about the eyes. Generalized aches. Malaise. Fever. Inflammation of one or more of the sinuses, hollow cavities in the skull connected with the nasal cavity. May result from colds and other upper respiratory infections, dental infection, allergy.

WHAT TO DO
- **Consult your physician.**
- Steam inhalation promotes needed drainage. May be treated with antibiotics.

TONSILLITIS

SYMPTOMS

Sore throat. Throat pain, especially on swallowing, often extending to the ears. Fever to 105° or 106°F./40.5° or 41.1°C. Chills. Malaise. Headache. Vomiting. Acute inflammation of the tonsils, the two lymph tissue masses in the sides of the throat, behind and above the tongue.

WHAT TO DO
- **Consult your physician.**
- Most cases of acute tonsillitis are due to bacteria and respond well to antibiotic treatment. Rest and warm salt water gargles help relieve discomfort. In viral tonsillitis, they are the only useful measures, since antibiotics do not affect viruses.
- Repeated attacks of acute tonsillitis or persistence of chronic tonsillitis and sore throat relieved only briefly by antibiotic treatment may call for tonsil removal.

TRAUMA TO THE NOSE

SYMPTOMS

Swelling. Tenderness. May result from a blow to the nose.

WHAT TO DO
- Prompt application of ice packs can help minimize swelling and control any bleeding; see **NOSE INJURIES: NOSEBLEED** in Part One.
- Consult your physician if there is any possibility of a fracture.

NUTRITIONAL DISORDERS

ALL-VEGETARIAN DIET DEFICIENCY

SYMPTOMS

May include: Anemia. Tongue inflammation. Sensations of numbness. Because vitamin B_{12}, which is essential for red blood cell formation, is not found in fruits and vegetables, vegans (pure vegetarians) who do not use milk or eggs may suffer from deficiency of the vitamin and resulting symptoms. Other vegetarians consuming milk and eggs do not have such problems.

WHAT TO DO
- The cause should be corrected through supplementary doses of vitamin B_{12}. Vegans also must take care to

get a proper mixture of fruits and vegetables in order to obtain all needed amino acid constituents of protein.
•Consultation with a nutritionist can be helpful.

DIETARY DEFICIENCIES IN PREGNANCY

SYMPTOMS

May include: Anemia. Fatigue. Breathlessness. The most recently revised (1980) Recommended Dietary Allowances of the Food and Nutrition Board, National Academy of Sciences — National Research Council indicate that women in pregnancy need 300 more calories a day than nonpregnant women of comparable weight and height.

WHAT TO DO

•Pregnancy calls for more than usual amounts of protein (meat, fish, eggs, fowl), calcium (skim or whole milk), iron (liver, kidney, whole wheat, raisins, dates, other foods).
•Consultation with a nutritionist can be helpful.

FOLIC ACID DEFICIENCY

SYMPTOMS

May include: Anemia. Infertility. Intestinal malabsorption. Inflamed tongue and mouth. The deficiency has been found associated with other conditions including skin disorders (psoriasis, rosacea, eczema), miscarriage and psychiatric disorders, although it has not been proved to cause them. Folic acid is found in many plant and animal tissues but may be destroyed by boiling or canning. Causes of the deficiency include: poor diet lacking fresh, only slightly cooked food; inadequate absorption or utilization resulting from alcoholism, celiac disease, sprue and the use of some drugs (phenytoin, primidone, barbiturates, oral contraceptives). Increased requirements — as during pregnancy and infancy — may also lead to a deficiency.

WHAT TO DO

•**Consult your physician.**
•Treatment includes administration of folic acid as needed and correction of the underlying cause of the deficiency when possible.

OBESITY

SYMPTOMS

Obvious excessive fat. Poor tolerance for exercise. Easy tiring. Sometimes: Increased tendency to arthritis, diabetes, high blood pressure. May possibly be attributable to genetic, glandular or other metabolic factors, but the vast majority of cases are caused by overeating in relation to the body's actual needs and expenditures.

WHAT TO DO

•A suitable diet is necessary along with increased exercise. Avoid fad diets. They produce quick losses, mostly of water. But they cannot be lived with for long, and there is a consequent regaining of weight. Perhaps the best diet is a well-balanced one, emphasizing only moderate caloric reduction, with limited amounts of the widest possible variety of foods. The objective should be to lose weight slowly, over a period of months. Once weight is stabilized at the desired point, the diet can be augmented a little for maintenance, and enjoyed thereafter. Consulting a nutritionist can be helpful.

SALT DEFICIENCY

SYMPTOMS

May include: Damp, cold skin. Stomach cramps. Muscle twitching. Sometimes: Convulsions. Actually, Americans get 2, 3 or even more times the amount of salt needed in the daily diet. But under some conditions such as vigorous exercise in very hot weather, large amounts of salt may be lost in perspiration, causing a deficiency.

WHAT TO DO

•For acute symptoms of deficiency, sip a mixture of about half a teaspoonful of salt dissolved in half a glass of water.

VITAMIN A DEFICIENCY

SYMPTOMS

In CHILDREN: Growth retardation. At ALL AGES: Greater susceptibility to infection. Night blindness. Sometimes: Abnormal dryness of the surface of the conjunctiva in the eye and softening of the cornea. Vitamin A is plentiful in many foods: liver, egg yolk, butter, cream, green leafy and yellow vegetables. Deficiency may occur, rarely in this country, from inadequate intake of vitamin A-rich foods. It also may result from interference with the body's absorption and storage, which can be caused by many diseases, including celiac syndrome, sprue, cystic fibrosis, ulcerative colitis, cirrhosis of the liver.

WHAT TO DO

•**Consult your physician.**
•The cause should be corrected. Therapeutic doses of vitamin A should immediately be taken, but only under medical supervision in order to avoid vitamin A toxicity.
•Consulting a nutritionist can be helpful.

VITAMIN A TOXICITY
(Hypervitaminosis A)

SYMPTOMS

May begin with: Coarse hair. Eyebrow loss. Dry, rough skin. Cracked lips. Later symptoms: Severe headache. Weakness. Joint pains. Liver and spleen enlargement. Results from taking excessive amounts of vitamin A.

WHAT TO DO

- Stop taking vitamin A immediately. Improvement usually occurs within 1 to 4 weeks.
- It may be advisable to consult your physician and a nutritionist.

VITAMIN B₁ (THIAMINE) DEFICIENCY
(Beriberi)

SYMPTOMS

Early symptoms: Fatigue. Irritability. Impaired memory. Disturbed sleep. Chest pain. Appetite loss. Abdominal discomfort. Constipation. Later symptoms may include: Abnormal sensations in the toes. Sensation of burning feet. Calf muscle cramps. Pains in the legs. Breathing difficulty. Occurs in people living largely on a diet of highly polished rice, which does not supply an adequate amount of the vitamin. May result from increased needs required by hyperthyroidism, pregnancy, fever. Can also be caused by impaired absorption (as in diarrhea) or impaired use (as in liver disease). May occur in alcoholism because of a combination of factors — decreased intake, impaired absorption, increased need.

WHAT TO DO

- **Consult your physician.**
- Any underlying cause should be corrected. Treatment will include suitable thiamine doses, 10 to 100 milligrams a day, depending on the need.
- Consulting a nutritionist can be helpful.

VITAMIN B₂ (RIBOFLAVIN) DEFICIENCY

SYMPTOMS

Dry scaling and fissuring of the lips and angles of the mouth. Sometimes: Red, scaly greasy areas on the ears, eyelids, scrotum and labia majora. Eye disturbances including light sensitivity and tearing. May result from inadequate intake of milk or other animal proteins containing the vitamin or because of chronic diarrhea, liver disease or alcoholism.

WHAT TO DO

- **Consult your physician.** Diagnosis is necessary because some symptoms may result from other problems including vitamin B₆ deficiency.
- In treatment, riboflavin may be given in divided doses of 10 to 30 milligrams a day until improvement occurs. Any underlying cause will be corrected if possible.
- Consulting a nutritionist can be helpful.

VITAMIN B₃ (NIACIN, NICOTINIC ACID) DEFICIENCY (Pellagra)

SYMPTOMS

May include any or many of the following: Abdominal discomfort. Nausea. Vomiting. Diarrhea. Bright scarlet tongue and mouth membranes. Sore mouth. Swollen tongue. Redness, blistering and crusting of the skin, and other skin disturbances. Excitation. Depression. Impaired memory. Confusion. Disorientation. May result from a major reliance on corn in the diet, a diarrheal disease, alcoholism, cirrhosis of the liver.

WHAT TO DO

- **Consult your physician.** The vitamin deficiency must be distinguished from other possible causes of similar symptoms.
- In treatment, upward of 300 milligrams a day in divided doses may be prescribed.
- Consulting a nutritionist can be helpful.

VITAMIN C (ASCORBIC ACID) DEFICIENCY (Scurvy)

SYMPTOMS

May begin with: Lassitude. Irritability. Weakness. Weight loss. Vague joint and muscle pains. Later symptoms may include: Swollen gums. Loosened teeth. Old scars break down. New wounds fail to heal. Spontaneous bleeding. In infants, may be due to lack of supplementary vitamin C. In adults, can be due to poor diet, gastrointestinal disease, thyroid disease, or pregnancy and nursing, which increase the need for the vitamin.

WHAT TO DO

- **Consult your physician.** In infants, the deficiency must be distinguished from rickets, rheumatic fever and other diseases which may produce similar symptoms. In adults, must be distinguished from arthritis, bleeding diseases and other conditions.
- In treatment, suitable doses of ascorbic acid will be prescribed according to age and need. Underlying problems, if any, will also be treated.
- Consulting a nutritionist can be helpful.

VITAMIN D DEFICIENCY
(Rickets, osteomalacia)

SYMPTOMS

In INFANTS, symptoms of rickets may include: **Restlessness. Poor sleeping. Bone softening. Bone bending. Misshapen skull. Bowleg. Knock-knee. In ADULTS, symptoms of osteomalacia (demineralization): Bone softening, particularly in the spine, pelvis and legs. Bowleg. Vertebrae shorten vertically.** Both rickets and osteomalacia result from inadequate exposure to sunlight, inadequate dietary intake and malabsorption or poor utilization of the vitamin.

WHAT TO DO

- **Consult your physician.** Vitamin D deficiency must be distinguished from other possible causes of similar symptoms, including severe thyroid deficiency in infants, hyperparathyroidism and other disorders in adults.
- Treatment is with suitable doses of vitamin D and, if necessary, calcium and phosphorus.
- Consulting a nutritionist can be helpful.

VITAMIN D TOXICITY
(Hypervitaminosis D)

SYMPTOMS

Appetite loss. Nausea. Vomiting. Excessive urination. Excessive thirst. Weakness. Nervousness. Itching. Results from excessive vitamin D intake. The toxicity can be dangerous, producing kidney damage that may be irreversible.

WHAT TO DO

- **Consult your physician.**
- In addition to immediate discontinuance of the vitamin, treatment includes a low-calcium diet and measures to keep the urine acid.
- Consulting a nutritionist can be helpful.

VITAMIN K DEFICIENCY

SYMPTOMS

Blood fails to clot normally. Either slow bleeding from the nose, gums, stomach or other areas, or massive bleeding into the gastrointestinal tract. Vitamin K, which is required for normal clotting, is obtained primarily from bacteria that produce it in the intestinal tract. Green leafy vegetables are also sources. The deficiency can result from reduction of the bacteria by antibacterial drugs used to fight infection; use of mineral oil as a laxative, which interferes with the absorption of the vitamin; ulcerative colitis, sprue, celiac disease and other gastrointestinal disorders that may cause malabsorption.

WHAT TO DO

- **Consult your physician.**
- Treatment includes administering suitable doses of vitamin K and correcting the underlying cause of the deficiency.
- Consulting a nutritionist can be helpful.

PARASITES: EXTERNAL

CRAB LOUSE

SYMPTOMS

Itching in the anogenital area. Tiny dark brown specs (louse excreta) on undergarments. Sometimes: Lice may be visible as small bluish spots on the skin of the trunk. Usually transmitted by sexual contact.

WHAT TO DO

- **Consult your physician.**
- Treatment with the prescribed medication usually produces cure within 2 days.

HEAD LOUSE INFESTATION

SYMPTOMS

Severe itching of the scalp, sometimes of the eyebrows and eyelashes. The infestation (pediculosis capitis) is transmitted by personal contact, combs, hats. Common among schoolchildren.

WHAT TO DO

- **Consult your physician.**
- Cure is rapid with a prescribed medicated shampoo.

SCABIES ("The itch")

SYMPTOMS

Itching, most intense when in bed. Mostly on finger webs, wrists, elbows, underarms, breasts, genitals and along the beltline. Caused by the itch mite Sarcoptes scabiei, which burrows into the skin and deposits its eggs. Can be transmitted through a family by skin-to-skin contact, but not by clothing or bedding.

WHAT TO DO

- Consult your physician.
- Cure can be obtained with a prescribed medicated cream or lotion.

TICKS

SYMPTOMS

Bites of some ticks may produce: Appetite loss.

Lethargy. Muscle weakness. Incoordination. Sometimes: Paralysis. Bites of others may produce: Blisters that fill with pus, then rupture and ulcerate. Local swelling. Pain.

WHAT TO DO

- Consult your physician.
- Treatment of tick paralysis may require administration of oxygen, respiratory stimulants, other measures. The tick lesions require cleaning.

PARASITES: INTERNAL

AFRICAN SLEEPING SICKNESS (Trypanosomiasis)

SYMPTOMS

Begin with: Irregular fever. Enlarged lymph nodes. Skin eruptions. Later symptoms: Tremors. Headache. Apathy. Convulsions which may lead to coma and death. A chronic disease caused by protozoa of the genus Trypanosoma, spread by tsetse fly bite. Virtually never occurs in the U.S.

WHAT TO DO

- Consult your physician.
- Treated with prescribed medication.

AMEBIC DYSENTERY

SYMPTOMS

Diarrhea. Stools that may contain blood and mucus. Slight fever. Recurrent cramps. Weight loss. Fatigue. Caused by invasion of the intestine by an amebic parasite, Entamoeba histolytica. A tropical disease that sometimes breaks out in epidemics in the U.S. Transmitted by sewage-contaminated water, flies, insects, infected food handlers.

WHAT TO DO

- Consult your physician.
- Treated with prescribed medication.

BILHARZIASIS (Schistosomiasis)

SYMPTOMS

Begin with: An outbreak of itching skin at the site where the parasites enter the body. Later symptoms may include: Fever. Hives. Liver and spleen enlargement. Lymph node swelling. Chronic diarrhea. Caused by infection with blood flukes coming from freshwater snails. The blood flukes swim freely and can penetrate the skin upon contact when the person is swimming or wading. The disease is common in Africa, the Middle East, Cyprus, some islands of the West Indies, northern areas of South America, Japan, some areas of China, the Philippines.

WHAT TO DO

- Consult your physician.
- An antimony-based compound and other medication may be used in treatment.

HOOKWORM DISEASE

SYMPTOMS

An itching rash may appear where hookworm larvae penetrate the skin, usually on the sole of a foot. Other symptoms may include: Upper abdominal pain. Darkening of stool with blood pigments. Iron-deficiency anemia. Retarded growth. Hookworm disease, particularly common in the southern part of the U.S., results from walking barefoot in fecally contaminated soil.

WHAT TO DO

- Consult your physician.
- Treatment may include iron therapy for the anemia and anti-hookworm medication.

MALARIA

SYMPTOMS

Abrupt chilly sensation or shaking chill. Fever. Sweats. Periodic attacks of chills and fever may follow. Other symptoms may include: Severe headache. Drowsiness. Appetite loss. Fatigue. Delirium. Confusion. Caused by a mosquito-transmitted parasite, Plasmodium. Occurs mostly in the tropics.

WHAT TO DO

- Consult your physician.

- Treated with an antimalarial drug.
- Medication can be prescribed to protect travelers to malarious areas.

PINWORM INFECTION

SYMPTOMS

Itching around the anal area. The tiny pinworm is the most common parasite among children in temperate climates. Infestation results from transfer of eggs from the anal area to the mouth and to toilet seats, clothing and bedding. Airborne eggs may also be inhaled or swallowed.

WHAT TO DO

- Pinworm infestation can be detected by finding the female worm in the anal area 1 or 2 hours after a child has been put to bed at night.
- **Consult your physician.**
- A single oral dose of prescribed medication can eradicate the infestation.
- Treatment for all members of the family may be advisable.

ROUNDWORM INFECTION

SYMPTOMS

Colicky abdominal pains. Diarrhea. A large parasite, the roundworm looks somewhat like an earthworm. It can grow up to 15 inches long. Its eggs enter the body through fecal-contaminated water, food and hands.

WHAT TO DO

- **Consult your physician.**
- Can be treated effectively with prescribed medication.

TAPEWORM

SYMPTOMS

There may be no symptoms. The only sign of infestation may be worm segments in stools. In some cases, symptoms may include one or more of the following: Pain about the stomach area. Diarrhea. Weight loss. Muscle pains. Weakness. Fever. Tapeworms of various kinds can measure from 8 to 15 feet in length when full-grown. Infestation stems from eating uncooked or improperly cooked beef, pork or freshwater fish containing tapeworm larvae.

WHAT TO DO

- **Consult your physician.**
- Can be treated effectively with a single oral dose of prescribed medication.

TOXOPLASMOSIS

SYMPTOMS

Symptoms of the more common MILD form: Swelling of the neck and underarm lymph nodes. Malaise. Muscle pain. Irregular mild fever. Mild anemia. Symptoms of the ACUTE form may include: Rash. High fever. Chills. Prostration. Symptoms of the CHRONIC form may include: Muscular weakness. Headache. Diarrhea. Weight loss. Eye inflammation. Symptoms of the CONGENITAL form, appearing soon after birth or months or years later, apparently as a result of infection in the mother during pregnancy, may include: Eye, central nervous system and other disturbances. Convulsions. Sometimes: Blindness. Mental retardation. The small protozoan parasite responsible is usually transmitted by exposure to cat feces containing the organism. It may also be transmitted by eating raw or undercooked contaminated meat.

WHAT TO DO

- **Consult your physician immediately.** Early treatment is important.
- Treatment may include prescribed medication.

TRICHINOSIS

SYMPTOMS

An early symptom: Swelling of the upper eyelids. May be followed by: Retinal hemorrhage. Eye pain. Sensitivity to light. Other symptoms may occur soon after: Muscle soreness and pain. Hives. Thirst. Profuse sweating. Fever. Chills. Weakness. Prostration. Possible later symptoms: Lymph node swellings. Encephalitis. Meningitis. Caused by a roundworm, Trichinella spiralis, transmitted by eating insufficiently cooked pork or pork products.

WHAT TO DO

- **Consult your physician.**
- Treatment may include bed rest and prescribed medication. In most cases, treatment is effective.

REPRODUCTIVE SYSTEM: FEMALE

AMENORRHEA
(Absence of menstruation)

SYMPTOMS

Failure to menstruate. May be **PRIMARY,** when menstruation fails to appear in a girl at least 16 years of age. Or may be **SECONDARY,** when menstruation ceases in a woman who has menstruated before. Amenorrhea may result from anatomic abnormalities (of the vagina, uterus or ovaries) or endocrine disorders (of the pituitary, thyroid or ovaries). Among many other possible causes: nutritional disturbances, effects of drugs such as barbiturates, opiates, corticosteroids, phenothiazines.

WHAT TO DO
- **Consult your physician.**
- Thorough physical examination and laboratory studies are required. Treatment is for the cause.

CERVICITIS

SYMPTOMS

After coitus, may include: Vaginal discharge. Vaginal bleeding. Heavy menstrual flow. Discomfort. Pain. Inflammation of the cervix, the lower end of the uterus extending into the vagina.

WHAT TO DO
- **Consult your physician.**
- Treatment may involve cauterization or in some cases dilation and curettage to remove infected tissues.

CHRONIC CYSTIC MASTITIS
(Fibrocystic disease of the breast)

SYMPTOMS

Appearance of cysts, usually in both breasts, often multiple and of many sizes. May give breasts a "cobblestone" feel. Sometimes with: Tenderness. Premenstrual discomfort. A benign condition, it is the most common disease of the breast, affecting about one-fifth of premenopausal women. The cause is not definitively established, but ovarian hormones may be involved.

WHAT TO DO
- **Consult your physician.**
- Treatment such as surgical removal is rarely required. But because women with fibrocystic disease have a 3 times greater risk than other women of developing breast cancer later in life, regular medical checkups are advisable.

CYSTOCELE AND RECTOCELE

SYMPTOMS

Muscles supporting the bladder and rectum may sometimes be stretched in childbirth and may lose their tone with lack of adequate physical exertion. In CYSTOCELE, because of the loss of firm muscular support, there may be stress incontinence, or loss of urine with sneezing, coughing, laughing or straining. In RECTOCELE, because of the loss of support, the rectum may sag and cause difficulty with bowel movement.

WHAT TO DO
- **Consult your physician.**
- Until childbearing is completed, relief may be obtained by use of a pessary, or plastic ring, inserted into the vagina to prevent protrusion of the bladder or rectum. Later, a plastic repair operation within the vagina may be recommended to tighten the supporting muscles.

ENDOMETRIOSIS

SYMPTOMS

May include any or many of the following: Pelvic pain. Painful menstruation. Excessive menstruation. Sterility. Painful intercourse. Presence of tissue like that of the mucous membrane of the uterus in the ovaries or other sites such as the abdomen.

WHAT TO DO
- **Consult your physician.**
- Treatment depends on age, severity of symptoms, desire to have children and other factors. Pregnancy often inhibits endometriosis and may be tried. In some cases, hormone therapy may be prescribed to relieve symptoms. Surgery may be recommended.

FIBROID TUMORS
(Myoma of the uterus)

SYMPTOMS

May include: Painful menstruation. Abnormal menstrual bleeding. Vaginal discharge. Frequent urination. Myomas — benign tumors of the smooth muscle fibers of the uterus — occur in more than 25 percent of women over age 35. Although a single tumor may occur, usually there are several. Often they are small, but they may grow large and occupy much of the uterine wall. Growth usually stops after menopause.

WHAT TO DO
- **Consult your physician.**
- When small, only periodic checking may be needed. For larger tumors causing significant symptoms, surgery may be recommended.

FRIGIDITY

SYMPTOMS

Inability to derive pleasure and satisfaction from sex. Can range from total disinterest to varying degrees of inadequate response to stimulation. May involve emotional factors, physical causes or both. Emotional factors include inadequate stimulation, marital discord, stressful life situations and depression or other psychiatric disturbances. Among the physical causes are thyroid disorder, diabetes mellitus, muscular disorders, effects of drugs such as oral contraceptives, antihypertensives and tranquilizers.

WHAT TO DO

- **Consult your physician.**
- If a physical disorder is involved, it should be treated. Emotional or sexual counseling may be helpful and may need to include both partners.

GERMAN MEASLES (RUBELLA) IN PREGNANCY

SYMPTOMS

Begin with: Malaise. Lymph node swelling behind the ears and in back of the neck. Fever. Slight cold and sore throat. Progress to: A light rose-colored rash on the face and neck that quickly spreads to the trunk and extremities. A flush may also appear, particularly on the face. The rash usually lasts about 3 days. Rubella contracted during pregnancy can be hazardous to the fetus. The congenital malformation rate is 10 to 50 percent when the mother has rubella in the first month of pregnancy, up to 25 percent in the second month, up to 17 percent in the third month. Rubella during the fourth, fifth and sixth months may result in fetal death or congenital abnormalities, but the rate is not known. Among common fetal defects are cataracts, deafness and heart disease.

WHAT TO DO

- **Consult your physician immediately.**
- Immune serum globulin may be given to a pregnant woman who has been exposed to rubella if blood testing within 7 days of exposure reveals no evidence of infection. If infection is present, interruption of pregnancy may be considered.

INFERTILITY

SYMPTOMS

Inability to become pregnant. Infertility is present in about 10 percent of American marriages. In about 40 percent of the cases, there is a male deficiency, in 20 percent a female hormonal defect, in 30 percent a female tubal disorder and in 10 percent a cervical environment that militates against fertility.

WHAT TO DO

- **Consult your physician.** A check of both husband and wife is essential.
- Treatment will be for cause. If ovulation or egg release is impaired, medication may be prescribed. For a uterine abnormality, surgery may be recommended.

MENOPAUSE

SYMPTOMS

In some cases: None. In other cases, one or more of the following: **Hot flushes. Sweating. Headache. Emotional instability. Appetite loss. Dyspepsia. Puffiness. Fatigue. Crying.** When ovulation and menstruation cease and the female hormones are diminished, there is a period of adjustment for the body, during which symptoms may or may not arise.

WHAT TO DO

- **For severe symptoms, consult your physician.**
- In some cases, estrogen may be used in minimal doses for a brief period. Other medication may be prescribed if needed.

MISCARRIAGE (Spontaneous abortion)

SYMPTOMS

Delivery or loss of the fetus during the first 20 weeks of pregnancy. Heralded by: Bleeding. Cramping. About 30 to 40 percent of women experience bleeding or cramping during the first 20 weeks and 20 percent actually miscarry. In many cases, the aborted fetus is found to be malformed, suggesting that miscarriage sometimes may be nature's way of interrupting the development of a defective fetus. Other possible causes of miscarriage include an incompetent or torn cervix, abnormalities of the uterus, hypothyroidism, diabetes mellitus, chronic kidney disease, infection, severe emotional shock.

WHAT TO DO

- **Consult your physician.**
- A threatened miscarriage sometimes may be treated by bed rest, which often reduces bleeding and cramping, and by avoiding intercourse. Hormones sometimes may be used, although there is evidence that they help in only a few instances. If the cervix is incompetent, its correction may help.
- If the miscarriage occurs, it should be completed by a physician.

MORNING SICKNESS

SYMPTOMS

Nausea in the early weeks of pregnancy.

WHAT TO DO

- **Consult your physician.**
- Drinking and eating only small amounts at a time may help. Soda crackers and a soft drink often relieve the nausea. If severe morning sickness continues, medication may be prescribed.

ORGASMIC FAILURE

SYMPTOMS

Failure to have an orgasm. Emotional or physical causes may be involved. See **FRIGIDITY.**

WHAT TO DO
- Consult your physician.
- If a physical disorder is involved, it requires treatment. Emotional or sexual counseling may be helpful and may need to include both partners.

OVARIAN TUMOR

SYMPTOMS

May begin with: Vague lower abdominal discomfort. Mild digestive complaints. Progress to: Swollen abdomen. Pelvic pain. Some tumors produce menstrual irregularities. Some are masculinizing, causing: Early cessation of menstruation. Deep voice. Hairiness. About 1 in 4 tumors removed surgically proves to be cancerous.

WHAT TO DO
- Consult your physician.
- Surgery is usually recommended.

PAINFUL INTERCOURSE AND VAGINAL SPASM
(Dyspareunia, vaginismus)

SYMPTOMS

Painful or difficult intercourse, with pain occurring during or following coitus. DYSPAREUNIA, which means painful intercourse, may sometimes be due to VAGINISMUS, a spasm of the lower vaginal muscles. Causes of both dyspareunia and vaginismus may be similar: local injury such as tears of the hymen, bruising of the urethra, inadequate lubrication (often due to improper or insufficient foreplay), inflammation or infection, allergic reactions to contraceptive foams, jellies, etc. Psychological factors such as fear of pregnancy, excessive modesty, aversion to intercourse may play a role.

WHAT TO DO
- Consult your physician.
- Treatment includes correction of any underlying physical causes. In vaginismus, graduated dilation often helps. A soothing ointment may be prescribed for any injuries. Liberal use of a lubricant just before intercourse may be helpful. Sexual or psychiatric counseling may sometimes be needed.

PAINFUL MENSTRUATION
(Dysmenorrhea)

SYMPTOMS

Mild to severe cramplike pain, usually in the lower abdomen, sometimes in the thighs or back, beginning just before or during menstruation, persisting for a few hours or through the entire period. Often with: Frequent urination. Nausea. Diarrhea. Backache. Headache. Sometimes: Distended abdomen. Painful breasts. PRIMARY DYSMENORRHEA begins soon after puberty and may be associated with uterine development, hormonal changes or emotional factors. SECONDARY DYSMENORRHEA, beginning later in life, usually has physical causes such as myomas, polyps, inflammatory disease.

WHAT TO DO
- Consult your physician.
- Typically, primary dysmenorrhea ends with the first pregnancy. Medication may be prescribed.
- Secondary dysmenorrhea may be relieved symptomatically by the same drugs used for the primary form — and by treatment for the cause, which may involve antibiotics for inflammation, surgery for myoma or other problems.

PREGNANCY: MINOR DISORDERS

The body changes that take place during pregnancy may give rise to certain minor discomforts. (They are "minor" in the sense that they do not seriously threaten either the mother or child.) Many are relatively common and include:

BACKACHE. May stem from postural imbalance because of increasing weight of the abdomen or stretching of uterine ligaments. Often helpful: use of low-heeled shoes.

MILD SHORTNESS OF BREATH. The fetus' consumption of iron may diminish the oxygen-carrying hemoglobin in the mother's red blood cells. If bothersome, consult your physician for possible increase in iron supplementation. Consulting a nutritionist can be helpful.

CONSTIPATION, BELCHING, HEARTBURN. Constipation is due to pressure from the enlarging uterus against the lower colon and rectum. Avoid cathartics. It may help to drink more fluids and add more fiber to the diet (whole grain cereals, fruits, vegetables). Consulting a nutritionist can be helpful. Heartburn and belching may result from a delay in the stomach's emptying time. If bothersome, consult your physician.

HEMORRHOIDS. Pregnancy causes increased pressure on the vein system and may lead to hemorrhoids or exacerbate existing ones. Commonly, improvement occurs after delivery. Compresses help. Managing constipation is also helpful; see above. Also see HEMORRHOIDS.

VARICOSE VEINS. Pregnancy tends to increase pressure in the leg veins. Elastic stockings help; they should be put on before standing up in the morning.

PREMENSTRUAL TENSION

SYMPTOMS

Starting 7 to 10 days before menstruation: Body puffiness. Breast discomfort. Irritability. Nervousness. Headache. Depression. The symptoms disappear a few hours after the menstrual flow begins. The symptoms appear to be related to hormone fluctuations and the tendency of estrogen to retain fluids in the body.

WHAT TO DO

• For mild symptoms, no treatment may be indicated.
• **For more severe symptoms, consult your physician.** Limiting salt intake and use of a diuretic drug 24 to 36 hours before symptoms are expected may be recommended to relieve fluid retention.

PROLAPSED UTERUS

SYMPTOMS

May include: Lower abdominal cramps. Vaginal pain. Vaginal discharge. Frequent urgent urination. Painful intercourse. Protrusion of the uterus through the vaginal orifice as a result of stretching and weakening of the muscles and ligaments holding the uterus in place. May be caused by congenital weakness, numerous pregnancies, age, excessive coughing, heavy lifting.

WHAT TO DO

• **Consult your physician.**
• For relief, a pessary inserted in the vagina as a support may be prescribed.
• For permanent correction, surgery may be recommended.

THE Rh FACTOR

SYMPTOMS

In a newborn infant: Severe anemia. Poor feeding. Seizures. Interrupted breathing during sleep. Eighty-five percent of people have a factor in their blood called Rh. There is no problem until a child is born to a mother who is Rh negative and father who is Rh positive. During the first pregnancy, the mother develops antibodies against the Rh factor. These develop too late to harm the first baby. But their presence in subsequent pregnancies can cause destruction of fetal red blood cells, causing anemia and other symptoms.

WHAT TO DO

• If an infant is born with the Rh problem, a pediatrician should be ready to do a complete exchange tranfusion of blood.
• The Rh problem can be prevented by a vaccine given to the mother within 72 hours after delivery of the first baby.

TUBAL PREGNANCY

SYMPTOMS

Usually begin shortly after the first missed period: Cramping pain. Spotting. Implantation of the fertilized egg in a fallopian tube instead of the uterus. In about half the cases, the cause is a previous infection of the tube. In others, the cause is unknown.

WHAT TO DO

• **Consult your physician.**
• Tests can confirm the tubal pregnancy. Surgery may be recommended. The uterine tube usually must be removed, occasionally along with the ovary on that side. That still leaves the other tube and ovary for future pregnancies.

VAGINITIS AND LEUKORRHEA
(Vaginal inflammation and vaginal discharge)

SYMPTOMS

A disturbing, often whitish, nonbloody vaginal discharge. Excessive discharge (leukorrhea), with or without an odor, may indicate an abnormality. A yellow, white or creamy-white discharge may indicate infection of the vagina, cervix or uterine lining. A thick yellow discharge may mean gonorrhea. A frothy discharge may indicate infection by Trichomonas vaginalis, a protozoon. If the frothy discharge is also foul-smelling, there may also be infection with Candida, a yeastlike fungus. A foul discharge may indicate bacterial infection or a forgotten tampon, diaphragm or pessary. Other types of discharges also are possible.

WHAT TO DO

• **Consult your physician.**
• The specific cause must be determined. Sulfa drugs, antibiotics, antifungal or other measures may be prescribed.

REPRODUCTIVE SYSTEM: MALE

EPIDIDYMITIS

SYMPTOMS

Fever. Scrotal pain. Swollen scrotum. Inflammation of the epididymis, the spermatic cord where sperm are stored. Usually a complication of a prostate or other infection.

WHAT TO DO

• **Consult your physician.**

• Treatment may include bed rest, scrotal ice packs, medication for pain, antibiotics for the infection.

IMPOTENCE

SYMPTOMS

Inability to achieve or sustain normal erection. May be due to psychological or physical factors. A transient episode of erectile difficulty, experienced at some time by most men, may lead to anxiety and fear of failure which may maintain the impotence. Physical factors include diseases such as diabetes mellitus, underfunctioning of the pituitary or thyroid gland, alcoholism, drug dependence, multiple sclerosis, stroke, sometimes but not always surgery for the prostate, and drugs such as antihypertensives, tranquilizers, sedatives, amphetamines.

WHAT TO DO

• **Consult your physician.**
• Psychological impotence may respond to brief counseling. If necessary, sexual counseling using a special two-partner technique may be used. If physical factors are involved, they must be treated.

INFERTILITY

SYMPTOMS

Inability to fertilize the ovum. Infertility is common in men. It is responsible for 40 percent of total infertility among childless couples. Possible causes are many and include: impaired sperm production, which may be due to injury or infection of the testes, varicocele, reactions to drugs, thyroid or pituitary gland disorders; obstruction of the seminal tract, which may be due to congenital abnormalities, orchitis, epididymitis, prostatitis or other inflammations; impaired delivery of sperm into the vagina, which may be due to prostate removal, premature ejaculation or other causes.

WHAT TO DO

• **Consult your physician.**
• Careful diagnostic evaluation to pinpoint cause or causes is vital. Treatment then can often be effective.

ORCHITIS

SYMPTOMS

Swollen testes and scrotum. Pain. Fever. Inflammation of the testes as result of a blow, infection or mumps.

WHAT TO DO

• **Consult your physician.**
• Treatment may include bed rest, application of ice packs, medication for pain. If the orchitis is from infection, antibiotics may be prescribed.

PHIMOSIS

SYMPTOMS

Congenital or inflammatory constriction of the foreskin of the penis, which cannot be drawn back. May make erection painful.

WHAT TO DO

• **Consult your physician.**
• Surgery may be recommended.

PREMATURE EJACULATION

SYMPTOMS

Ejaculation of semen before or soon after the penis is inserted into the vagina. May result from inflammatory diseases such as those of the prostate or urethra (the canal extending from the bladder to outside the body). Emotional problems related to fear of failure may be involved.

WHAT TO DO

• **Consult your physician.**
• If an inflammatory disease is present, antibiotic or other treatment may be prescribed. Counseling of both partners by the physician or, if necessary, a sex therapist often is effective where fear of failure is involved.

PROSTATE ENLARGEMENT
(Benign prostatic hypertrophy)

SYMPTOMS

Progressively increasing frequent and urgent urination. Urination during the night. Hesitant and intermittent urinary stream. Dribbling. Sensation that the bladder has not been completely emptied. The enlarged prostate envelops the urethra, the canal that carries urine from the bladder, interfering with the normal urine flow. Common in men after 50. The cause is unknown.

WHAT TO DO

• **Consult your physician.**
• Surgery may be recommended.

PROSTATITIS

SYMPTOMS

In the ACUTE form: Chills. High fever. Frequent and urgent urination. Pain in the area between the scrotum and the anus and in the low back. Burning sensation on urinating. Sometimes: Joint pains. Muscle pains. Blood in the urine. In the CHRONIC form: Symptoms similar to those of the acute infection may develop, and in some cases the scrotum

may be affected with pain and swelling. An infection of the prostate.

- **Consult your physician.**
- Hospitalization may be necessary. Intensive therapy with antibiotics or other medication may be prescribed.

SCROTAL MASSES
(Hydrocele, spermatocele, varicocele)

SYMPTOMS

Swollen scrotum. A **HYDROCELE,** the most common mass, is a collection of fluid in the scrotum around the testes. A **SPERMATOCELE,** which resembles a hydrocele, is a cyst containing sperm, lying above a testis. A **VARICOCELE** is a collection of congested veins in the scrotum, sometimes but not always interfering with fertility.

WHAT TO DO

- **Consult your physician.** Any scrotal swelling should be checked and diagnosed professionally.
- If the mass is troublesome or cumbersome, surgery may be recommended. If it isn't, the physician may advise benign neglect.

UNDESCENDED TESTES

SYMPTOMS

Failure of one or both testes to descend completely into the scrotum before birth. May result from hormonal abnormalities or mechanical difficulties in the descent.

WHAT TO DO

- **Consult your physician.**
- If untreated, an undescended testis may show progressive failure of sperm production. Hormone treatment may be prescribed. Surgery may be recommended.

RESPIRATORY SYSTEM

ANTHRACOSIS (Black lung disease)

SYMPTOMS

Breathing difficulty. Coughing. Wheezing. Involves the deposit of coal dust throughout the lungs as a result of coal-mining. Because such symptoms may be produced by heavy cigarette smoking and most coal miners with the symptoms are heavy smokers, exactly how large a role coal dust plays in producing or aggravating the symptoms is not known.

WHAT TO DO

- **Consult your physician.**

ASBESTOSIS

SYMPTOMS

Gradual onset of breathing difficulty upon exertion. Reduced tolerance for exercise. Lung disorder caused by inhalation of asbestos fibers in mining, milling, manufacturing or application (as in insulation) of asbestos products. Leads to increased risk of lung cancer.

WHAT TO DO

- **Consult your physician.**
- Treatment may be similar to that for emphysema; see **EMPHYSEMA.**

ASPIRATION PNEUMONIA

SYMPTOMS

Fever. Coughing. Chest pains. Breathing difficulty. Pneumonia caused by foreign material accidentally breathed into the lungs. May occur after anesthesia, alcoholic intoxication, convulsive seizure or vomiting while not fully conscious.

WHAT TO DO

- **Consult your physician immediately.** Prompt treatment is important.
- As much of the foreign material as possible must be sucked up through a tube. Oxygen is usually given. Antibiotics and other medication may be prescribed.

ASTHMA

SYMPTOMS

Wheezing. Coughing. Shortness of breath. Pressure or tightness in the chest. Symptoms can differ greatly in severity and frequency from one patient to another. Reversible obstruction of the air passages. The cause is unknown. May be precipitated by different factors in different patients: viral respiratory infection, exercise, emotional upset, changes in temperature or barometric pressure, cold air, tobacco smoke, gasoline fumes or other irritants, allergy to pollens, molds, house dust or animal dander.

- **Consult your physician.**
- Medication may be prescribed to treat acute attacks and help reduce recurrences.

ATELECTASIS

SYMPTOMS

May include: Breathing difficulty. Bluish color. Drop in blood pressure. Racing pulse. Fever. Sometimes, the symptoms are mild. Shrunken, airless state of all or part of a lung. In **NEWBORNS,** may occur because of prematurity and failure of the lungs to expand at birth because of sticky lung secretions. In **OTHER CASES,** stems from airway obstruction caused by sticky secretions, foreign bodies, tumors, or lymph nodes pressing on the air passages.

WHAT TO DO

- **Consult your physician.**
- For newborn atelectasis, treatment may include suctioning of the windpipe to open the airway, administration of oxygen, measures to stimulate breathing and crying.
- In other cases, treatment may include eliminating the cause, stimulating coughing (sometimes with cough-inducing equipment), suctioning, and antibiotics for the infection.

ATYPICAL PNEUMONIA
("Viral pneumonia")

SYMPTOMS

May sometimes resemble those of the common cold. In other cases: Headache. Fever. Chilliness. Malaise. Severe coughing. Sputum containing mucus and pus, sometimes tinged with blood. Muscle pains. An inflammation or infection of the lungs. May be caused by viruses or by other organisms called Mycoplasma.

WHAT TO DO

- **Consult your physician.**
- Treatment may include bed rest, administration of oxygen if necessary, steam inhalation, medication. If caused by Mycoplasma, an antibiotic may be prescribed.

BRONCHIECTASIS

SYMPTOMS

Chronic coughing. Chronic sputum production. Typically the coughing occurs in a pattern — in the morning, late in the afternoon, on retiring, often with little or no coughing in between. **Coughing of blood is frequent. In severe cases: Breathing difficulty on exertion. Repeated respiratory infections may occur.** A chronic dilation of the air passages. In a few cases, the cause is congenital. Most often develops early in childhood after a severe pneumonia, particularly after one complicating a case of measles or whooping cough.

WHAT TO DO

- **Consult your physician.**
- Treatment is aimed at controlling the infection. May include antibiotics and postural drainage. In some cases, when the disease is well-localized, surgery may be recommended.

BRONCHITIS

SYMPTOMS

In the ACUTE form: Sore throat. Runny nose. Chilliness. Fever. Back pain. Muscle pain. Dry cough that changes to produce increasing amounts of sputum. An inflammation of the air passages. May follow a cold or other upper respiratory infection. Most common in winter. **The CHRONIC form begins with: Slight coughing, often present for years, that intensifies with colds. Other upper respiratory infections. Later: Increased sputum production. Breathing difficulty. Wheezing. Bluish color. Sometimes: Coughing paroxysms.** Chronic inflammation of the airways from cigarette smoking, air pollution or both. Involves degenerative changes adversely affecting the activity of cilia, the tiny hairlike processes in the airways which normally wave up bacteria and foreign matter to aid elimination.

WHAT TO DO

- **Consult your physician.**
- For acute bronchitis, treatment may include rest until fever subsides, fluids, steam inhalations, antibiotics and other medication.
- For chronic bronchitis, treatment may include elimination of smoking, avoiding irritants, using steam inhalations, postural drainage, regular exercise, antibiotics and other medication.

COMMON COLD: SEE COMMON COLD UNDER NOSE & THROAT.

EDEMA OF THE LUNGS
(Pulmonary edema)

SYMPTOMS

Extreme breathing difficulty. Bluish color. Sense of suffocation. Pallor. Profuse perspiration. Filling of the lungs with fluid. Most often results from heart disease. Other causes: lung infection, injury from chemical irritants.

WHAT TO DO
- **Seek medical aid immediately. Pulmonary edema can be life-threatening.**
- Treatment may include having the patient sit up with his legs dangling, administration of oxygen, intravenous medication, diagnosis and treatment of the cause.

EMPHYSEMA

SYMPTOMS

Wheezing. Labored breathing with even mild exertion. Chronic hard coughing. Thick sputum. A chronic disease in which the air spaces of the lung become distended and undergo destructive changes, making it difficult to exhale. Smoking is believed to be a major cause; air pollution may be another factor.

WHAT TO DO
- **Consult your physician.**
- Although emphysema cannot be cured, its symptoms can be relieved, potentially fatal exacerbations controlled, and progression of the disease slowed. Treatment may include antibiotics, bronchodilator drugs to enlarge the airways, expectorants and liquefying agents to help remove mucus and other obstructing materials, postural drainage, breathing exercises, other prescribed regular exercise, elimination of smoking.

EMPYEMA

SYMPTOMS

Chest pain on one side. Coughing. Fever. Chills. Breathing difficulty. Presence of pus in the fluid between the membrane layers enveloping a lung. May develop as a complication of pleurisy or other respiratory disease.

WHAT TO DO
- **Consult your physician.**
- Treatment may include rest, antibiotics, drainage with a tube to eliminate the pus collection.

FOREIGN BODY IN THE BRONCHI

SYMPTOMS

A breathed-in foreign object — food, loose dental filling, bone, etc. — may first cause choking and gagging until it passes into the bronchi. Symptoms then may stop, falsely suggesting that the object has been swallowed or eliminated. Later, an infection may develop, producing: Fever. Coughing.

WHAT TO DO
- **Consult your physician.**
- Usually treated by removing the object with a bronchoscope — a long tube.

HIGH ALTITUDE LUNG EDEMA

SYMPTOMS

Shortness of breath. Bluish color. Severe coughing, sometimes with blood. May be caused by a rapid ascent to a high altitude coupled with exertion.

WHAT TO DO
- **Consult your physician.**
- Meanwhile, immediately bring the victim down to a lower altitude. Administration of oxygen may be needed.

HYPERVENTILATION (Overbreathing)

SYMPTOMS

May produce any or many of the following: Faintness. Giddiness. Lightheadedness. Chest tightness. Smothering sensation. Heart pounding. Throat fullness. Pain over the stomach region. Muscle twitching. Cramps. Hyperventilation — abnormally prolonged and deep breathing, usually done unconsciously — leads to excessive loss of carbon dioxide in the expired air, causing respiratory alkalosis. May result from acute anxiety or emotional tension.

WHAT TO DO
- Symptoms can be relieved — and the role of overbreathing demonstrated — by rebreathing from a paper bag so the expired carbon dioxide is replaced.

HYPOXIA (Mountain sickness)

SYMPTOMS

Shortness of breath. Difficulty concentrating. Restlessness. Heart pounding. Nausea. Lip blueness. May occur in people unused to high altitudes who are suddenly exposed to it. Tolerance to high altitudes varies greatly. Some people are affected at 5,000 feet; others not until 10,000 feet or more.

WHAT TO DO
- Symptoms may gradually lessen after several days of acclimatization, during which physical effort should be minimized. If symptoms persist, oxygen and descent may be required.

LARYNGOTRACHEOBRONCHITIS (Croup)

SYMPTOMS

A child is often awakened at night by: Breathing dif-

ficulty. **"Barking" cough. Hoarseness. In severe cases: Bluish color may develop.** An acute viral inflammation of the respiratory tract, with swelling and obstruction. The child may appear improved in the morning but worsens again at night. Usually lasts 3 or 4 days.

WHAT TO DO

- **Consult your physician.** Croup should be distinguished from a foreign body or other infection.
- Home humidification may help. It can be administered by a vaporizer, humidifier or steam from a hot shower in a closed bathroom while the child is held on a parent's lap.
- If symptoms persist or worsen, hospitalization may be needed, with administration of oxygen, mist therapy, other measures.

LUNG ABSCESS

SYMPTOMS

Malaise. Appetite loss. Sweats. Chills. Fever. Coughing that may produce pus-laden sputum. Sometimes: Chest pain. May result from pneumonia, malignancy, foreign material getting into a lung during regurgitation.

WHAT TO DO

- **Consult your physician.**
- Treatment may include antibiotics, postural drainage, suction to remove thick sputum. In resistant cases, surgery may be recommended.

PLEURISY

SYMPTOMS

Sudden sharp, sticking pain in the chest. May be aggravated by breathing or coughing. Breathing is usually rapid and shallow. An inflammation of the pleura, the membrane investing the lungs. May result from injury to pleura, infection, complication of pneumonia.

WHAT TO DO

- **Consult your physician.**
- Treatment may include antibiotics, wrapping the chest with adhesive bandages to help relieve pain, medication, other measures as needed.

PNEUMONIA

SYMPTOMS

Sudden shaking chill. Fever to 105°F./40.5°C. Chest pain. Breathing difficulty. Dry hacking cough which later becomes loose and produces pinkish sputum that becomes rust-colored. Sweating. Bluish color. Sometimes: Abdominal distention. Diarrhea. Jaundice (skin yellowing). An acute infection of the lung which may be **LOBAR** (involving an entire lobe of a lung), **SEGMENTAL** (involving parts of the lobe only), **BRONCHIAL** (involving the airways). Caused by various microorganisms, including pneumococci, staphylococci, streptococci, Klebsiella, Haemophilus influenzae.

WHAT TO DO

- **Consult your physician immediately.**
- Treatment may include bed rest, antibiotics and other medication, fluids, oxygen if needed.

PNEUMOTHORAX (Collapsed lung)

SYMPTOMS

Sudden sharp chest pain. Breathing difficulty. Sometimes: Dry hacking cough. Pain may spread to the shoulder, across the chest or over the abdomen. It may sometimes mimic a heart attack. Results when air or gas gets between the membrane lining the chest wall and the membrane surrounding a lung, preventing the lung from expanding with each breath. May occur in the course of a lung disease or follow an injury to the chest wall.

WHAT TO DO

- **Consult your physician.**
- Treatment may include bed rest and oxygen for breathing difficulty. In some cases, air may be removed through a needle inserted in the chest.

SILICOSIS

SYMPTOMS

May include: Breathing difficulty, with deeper and more rapid breathing than normal. Sometimes: Dry coughing. In advanced cases: Malaise. Sleep disturbance. Appetite loss. Chest pain. Hoarseness. Bluish color. Coughing and spitting of blood. Lung disease from inhaling silica dust in mining, sandblasting tunnels, pottery making.

WHAT TO DO

- **Consult your physician.**
- No specific treatment is available. Improvement of symptoms may be achieved with drainage of bronchial secretions, medication, elimination of smoking to minimize irritation, prescribed exercise.

TUBERCULOSIS

SYMPTOMS

In early stages: Vary. Sometimes no symptoms. Sometimes fever and weight loss. In children, early TB may resemble a flu-like illness with: Fever. Appetite loss. Weight loss. Fatigue. Drowsiness. As disease progresses: Possible severe coughing.

Sputum becomes yellowish and often blood-streaked. Chest pain, aggravated by breathing. If leg bones and joints are affected: Joint pain. Swelling. Limping. If arms are affected: Joint swelling. Tenderness. Limitation of movement. If the spine is affected: Painful muscle spasm. Limitation of movement. Curvature of the spine. Abscess formation. A bacterial infection of the lungs, which may invade other parts of the body. May be transmitted from an infected person via droplets that are carried in the air or on eating utensils. May also be transmitted from infected cattle via unpasteurized milk and other dairy products.

WHAT TO DO

• **Consult your physician.**
• Treatment with prescribed medication is effective.

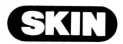

ABSCESS

SYMPTOMS

Painful, reddened area with accumulated pus. Caused by bacteria that invade by way of small wounds or breaks in the skin.

WHAT TO DO

• A small abscess may ''come to a head'' by itself, breaking through the skin and allowing the pus to drain. **Do not** squeeze the abscess; pressure on inflamed tissues is likely to spread the infection.
• **For a larger abscess, consult your physician.** Incision may be recommended. An antibiotic may be prescribed.

ACNE

SYMPTOMS

Blackheads, whiteheads, pimples, sometimes cysts on the face, neck, shoulders, chest, back. A common inflammatory disease affecting most teenagers and some adults. Involves an interaction between hormones, sebum (an oily sebaceous gland secretion needed for healthy skin) and bacteria. Often exacerbated in winter, improved in summer possibly because of beneficial effect of the sun.

WHAT TO DO

• In mild cases, washing the face several times a day with any good soap may be helpful if the skin is oily.
• **For moderate or severe acne, consult your physician.**
• Treatment may include antibiotics, application of vitamin A acid preparation, other measures.

ATHLETE'S FOOT

SYMPTOMS

May begin with: Dry scaling between the toes. **Followed by: Whitish, soggy, malodorous, itching lesions.** Begins as a fungus infection. Likely to occur with continued presence of moisture between the toes from sweating, swimming, etc. Later complicated by bacterial infection.

WHAT TO DO

• In early cases, daily bathing and thorough drying of the feet and application of Desenex or Tinactin may help.
• **For severe cases, consult your physician.** An antibiotic or other measures may be prescribed.

BALDNESS

SYMPTOMS

In MALE PATTERN BALDNESS, hair loss begins in front or over the crown of the head. If the loss starts in mid-teens, baldness eventually is often extensive. A familial condition. The cause is not entirely clear. In **TOXIC ALOPECIA,** another type of hair loss, the loss is temporary. May follow a severe feverish infection, the use of some drugs, overdoses of vitamin A, or may occur with a thyroid or pituitary gland disorder. In **ALOPECIA AREATA,** sudden hair loss occurs in small areas for no known reason, but the hair often reappears in a few months.

WHAT TO DO

• No treatment of any effectiveness is known for male pattern baldness.

BEDSORES (Decubitus ulcers)

SYMPTOMS

Begin with: Redness in bedridden patients on points of pressure such as heels, elbows, bony prominences. Later: Reddened areas break down and become ulcerated.

- Bedsores often represent a failure of good nursing care. A cardinal rule is to turn the patient every two hours to prevent bedsores from developing. This is a major help and often all that is needed. Also valuable: applying dusting powder or cornstarch.
- **For advanced cases, consult your physician immediately.** Medical treatment is urgent. It may include removal of dead tissue, application of medicated dressings, other measures.

BODY ODOR (Bromhidrosis)

SYMPTOMS

Excessive perspiration that is malodorous because of decomposition by bacteria and yeasts. Excessive sweating may sometimes result from a gland or nervous system disorder, but the cause mostly is unknown.

WHAT TO DO

- **Daily bathing and shaving the underarm hair are often helpful.**
- For extreme underarm sweating, surgical removal of some of the underarm sweat glands may be recommended.

BOILS AND CARBUNCLES

SYMPTOMS

A BOIL (furuncle) is an inflamed lump on and under the skin, filled with pus and with a central core. Most often occurs on the neck, breasts, face or buttocks. Most painful when it occurs on the nose, ear or fingers. A CARBUNCLE is a cluster of boils with a spread of infection under the skin. Occurs most often on the nape of the neck. Most frequent in men. Often accompanied by fever. Sometimes by prostration. In both boils and carbuncles, staphylococci are the most frequent causes of infection.

WHAT TO DO

- For a single boil, moist heat applications may induce pointing and spontaneous drainage.
- **Consult your physician** for a single boil on the nose or central facial area and for multiple boils and carbuncles. Antibiotics may be prescribed.

CONTACT DERMATITIS

SYMPTOMS

Redness. Itching. Blistering. Sometimes: Crustiness. An acute or chronic inflammation produced by substances that irritate or sensitize the skin. Any part of the skin in contact with the culprit substance may become involved. Among many possible causative substances: plants such as primrose, ragweed, chrysanthemum; chemicals such as mercury, chromates, pyrethrum; drugs such as antihistamines, tranquilizers, sulfa compounds, penicillin; household items such as polishes, detergents, waxes; fabrics such as silk, wool, synthetic fibers, leather, fur; cosmetics such as hair dyes, bleaches, deodorants.

WHAT TO DO

- **Consult your physician** unless you can identify the cause and remove it, and the dermatitis clears. Patch testing by the physician may help identify the cause.
- Treatment may include use of tap-water soaks or compresses to soothe the lesions. In severe cases, medication may be prescribed.

CORNS AND CALLUSES

SYMPTOMS

A CORN is a circumscribed, conical mass that causes pain by pressure on the nerve endings. One kind, the hard corn, is usually located on the outside of the little toe or on the upper surfaces of other toes. The soft corn, a white sodden mass, usually occurs between the fourth and fifth toes. A CALLUS is a localized area of skin thickening. It usually occurs on hands and feet but may occur in another area subject to excessive use. Corns are caused almost always by pressure or friction from tight shoes.

WHAT TO DO

- Corns often can be removed by soaking in warm water, then applying an agent such as 20 percent salicylic acid in collodion, covering with corn pads for several days, then soaking and removing. (Be careful not to apply the medication to the normal skin.)
- Calluses may be removed with salicylic acid plasters or a nail file or emery board.
- Soft, well-fitting shoes will help prevent recurrences. In some cases, it may also help to redistribute pressure with the aid of pads or rings, arch inserts or foam rubber protective pads.
- **For persons with diabetes or other circulatory disorders, consult your physician or chiropodist for proper foot care.**

DANDRUFF (Seborrheic dermatitis)

SYMPTOMS

Dry or greasy scaling of the scalp. Itching. In severe cases: Yellowish greasy scaling that may involve the hairline and other areas about the face and neck. The cause is unknown. Genetic and climatic factors may be involved; the condition tends to worsen in winter. Does not lead to hair loss.

WHAT TO DO
- A medicated shampoo is often effective.
- **For a severe case, consult your physician.** Medicated lotion, ointment or cream may be prescribed.

ERYSIPELAS

SYMPTOMS

Round or oval patches on the skin that enlarge and spread, then become red, tender and swollen. Chills. Fever. Sometimes: Nausea. Vomiting. An acute skin infection by streptococcal bacteria. Most often affects the face, arm or leg.

WHAT TO DO
- **Consult your physician.**
- Treatment may include antibiotics and other medication, cold packs for local relief.

HERPES SIMPLEX
(Cold sores, fever blisters)

SYMPTOMS

After a short period of itching or tingling, small tight blisters appear, most often on the lip or mouth, coalesce, persist for several days, dry, form a yellowish crust, usually heal completely within 3 weeks. A recurrent infection by herpes simplex, a virus. Can be triggered by sunlight, feverish illness, physical or emotional stress, some foods or drugs and, in many cases, by unknown factors.

WHAT TO DO
- Drying lotions or liquids such as camphor spirits or 70 percent alcohol may be helpful. Zinc oxide applied to crusts may speed recovery.

IMPETIGO

SYMPTOMS

Blisters on the face, arms or legs, which become filled with pus, break, become heavily crusted. A highly contagious skin infection usually caused by streptococcal bacteria, sometimes with staphylococci added. Occurs mainly in children.

WHAT TO DO
- **Consult your physician.**
- Treatment may include antibiotics, tap-water compresses.

LICHEN PLANUS

SYMPTOMS

Itching patches of violet-colored, pimple-like lesions, most often on the wrists, legs, trunk, glans penis, mouth and vaginal mucous membrane, only rarely the face. Seldom affects children. The cause is unknown, although some drugs such as arsenic, bismuth, gold and quinacrine may cause an eruption much like lichen planus. The first attack lasts for weeks or months, and there may be recurrences.

WHAT TO DO
- **Consult your physician.**
- If a cause is suspected, it will be removed. Treatment may include an antihistamine to decrease itching, other medication.

LUPUS ERYTHEMATOSUS

SYMPTOMS

In one form of the disease, CHRONIC DISCOID, limited to: A red eruption on the nose and cheek, somewhat resembling a butterfly. Itching. Scaling. The other, more serious form, SYSTEMIC, may also produce: Arthritis-like joint pains. Fever. Abdominal pain. Spleen enlargement. Of unknown cause. More frequent in women, most often during their 30s.

WHAT TO DO
- **Consult your physician.**
- For chronic discoid, treatment may include minimum exposure to sunlight, use of topical or oral medication.
- For the systemic form, medication may be prescribed.

MOLES AND BIRTHMARKS

SYMPTOMS

MOLES are fleshy skin growths or blemishes. They may be small or large; flat or raised; smooth, hairy or warty; black, yellow-brown or flesh colored. Mostly appear in childhood or adolescence; more sometimes appear during pregnancy. Everyone has at least a few. **BIRTHMARKS (angiomas) are blood vessel lesions. They include portwine stain, a flat, pink, red or purplish lesion; strawberry mark, a raised bright-red lesion which tends to increase slowly in size for several months, then disappear within 2 to 5 years; cavernous hemangioma, a raised red or purplish lesion; and lymphangioma, a raised, usually yellowish-tan but sometimes reddish lesion.** Birthmarks are either present at birth or appear shortly thereafter in about one-third of infants. Many disappear spontaneously; some persist.

- **Consult your physician for any mole that enlarges suddenly, darkens, shows spotty changes in color, bleeds, ulcerates or becomes inflamed and painful.** Such symptoms may indicate malignant melanoma. Removal may be recommended.
- Usually birthmarks require no treatment unless they are cosmetic handicaps or occur in areas (near the eye, for example) where they may interfere with function. Portwine stains are not treatable but often can be covered with a cosmetic cream. A strawberry mark may be treated with medication, surgery, dry ice, electrocoagulation or injection of a solution. A cavernous hemangioma may be treated with medication or electrocoagulation. For lymphangiomas, electrocoagulation or surgery may be recommended.

NEURODERMATITIS (Atopic dermatitis)

SYMPTOMS

Chronic itching. The skin is generally dry, without blisters or other lesions, but scratching and rubbing may cause outbreaks and skin thickening. A superficial skin inflammation. Usually occurs in people with a personal or family history of allergy. The cause is unknown.

WHAT TO DO

- **Consult your physician.**
- A medicated cream or ointment may be prescribed. Treatment may also include application of white petrolatum or hydrogenated vegetable cooking oil to help hydrate the skin, minimal bathing and use of soap on the affected area, bath oils to lubricate the skin.

PEMPHIGUS

SYMPTOMS

Clusters of large blisters, often occurring first in the mouth, where they rupture and remain as chronic, often painful erosions. Subsequently, similar blisters appear on the skin and leave raw, tender patches which later become crusted. A potentially grave disease of unknown cause. May be fatal unless adequately treated.

WHAT TO DO

- **Consult your physician immediately.** Hospitalization is usually required.
- Treatment may include antibiotics and other medication.

PITYRIASIS ROSEA

SYMPTOMS

Pinkish-oval patches on the trunk, sometimes on the arms. Often accompanied by itching. A mild inflammatory disease. Can occur at any age but most often affects young adults, with incidence highest in spring and autumn.

WHAT TO DO

- **Consult your physician.** Pityriasis should be differentiated from other skin diseases.
- Usually disappears within 4 or 5 weeks, and no treatment may be needed.
- Sunlight may hasten healing. Itching may be relieved by 0.25 percent menthol in a vanishing cream base. For severe itching, medication may be prescribed.

PSORIASIS

SYMPTOMS

Bright red patches covered with silvery scales, most often on the knees, elbows, scalp, chest, abdomen, backs of the arms and legs, palms, soles. The patches clear but then recur. Can occur at any age but most often appear between 10 and 40. The cause is unknown, but frequently there is a family history of psoriasis.

WHAT TO DO

- **Consult your physician.**
- Many forms of treatment can be used; some are helpful in some cases, others in other cases. They include lubricating creams, vegetable cooking oil or white petrolatum applied to the affected areas, alone or with added coal tar or medication. Other measures that may be useful include medicated ointment, nightly tar ointment application and daily exposure to sunlight. In severe, otherwise unresponsive cases, oral medication may be prescribed. Still other experimental treatments are under study.

RINGWORM

SYMPTOMS

Itching reddish patches, often blistered or scaly, sometimes becoming ring-shaped as the infection spreads. May affect the scalp, body, genital area, nails, areas between the toes. Caused by different types of fungi. Highly contagious. Spread by humans and animals, and on combs, towels or other objects handled by someone who is infected.

WHAT TO DO

- **Consult your physician.**
- Treatment may include use of antibiotics, medicated ointment, lotion or compresses.

ROSACEA

SYMPTOMS

Flushing of the skin of the nose, forehead, cheeks. Followed by: Reddening from dilation of tiny blood vessels. Acne-like pimples. Usually begins in middle age or later. The cause is unknown.

WHAT TO DO

- **Consult your physician.**
- An antibiotic may be prescribed.

SCLERODERMA (Hidebound skin, progressive systemic sclerosis)

SYMPTOMS

May begin with: Gradual thickening of the skin of the fingers. Joint pains. As the disease progresses: The skin of much or all of the body becomes tight and shiny. The face becomes masklike. May sometimes involve the gastrointestinal tract, lungs, kidneys and heart, producing: Heartburn. Regurgitation of food from the stomach to the esophagus. Malabsorption. High blood pressure. Pleurisy. Heart rhythm abnormalities. A chronic disease of unknown cause. Rare in children, it is more common in women than men. May occur in a mild form with no threat to life or a severe form that may shorten life.

WHAT TO DO

- **Consult your physician immediately.**
- Treatment may include antibiotics and other medication, blood vessel dilators, physiotherapy.

VITILIGO (Piebald skin)

SYMPTOMS

Milky white patches of skin that have lost pigmentation and are prone to sunburn. There may be only a few patches, or they may cover the entire body. The cause is unknown, although the disorder sometimes tends to run in families.

WHAT TO DO

- **Consult your physician.** In some cases, repigmentation has been reported after treatment.
- Cosmetic creams may be used to hide small patches. Aminobenzoic acid solution or gel protect against sunburn.

WARTS

SYMPTOMS

Usually, rough-surfaced, firm, round or irregular light gray, yellow, brown or grayish-black growths on the skin. Appear most often on the fingers, elbows, knees, face or scalp, but may spread elsewhere. PLANTAR WARTS on the sole are flattened by pressure and may be very tender. FILIFORM WARTS — long, narrow, small growths — occur on the eyelids, face, neck or lips. Caused by a virus. Benign but contagious. Occur most often in older children. May persist for years or disappear in months.

WHAT TO DO

- **Consult your physician** if warts are bothersome.
- Warts may be removed with various types of treatment: Freezing with liquid nitrogen, electrodessication, medicated application, salicylic acid plaster, paring.

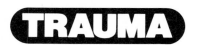

TRAUMA

HEAD INJURY

SYMPTOMS

In BRAIN CONCUSSION from a severe head injury, symptoms may include: Dizziness. Nausea. Weak pulse. Loss of consciousness. On regaining consciousness, there may be: **Severe headache. Blurred vision. In a CEREBRAL CONTUSION from a severe head injury, symptoms may include: Severe surface wounds. Fractures at the base of the skull. Labored breathing. Rigidly bent arms. Clenched jaw. The legs and often the trunk are extended. If HEMATOMA, a** tumor-like mass of coagulated blood, is present, symptoms may include one or more of the following: **Increasing headache. Inability to move normally. Dilated pupils. Coma.** Other symptoms which may result from severe head injury include: **Bleeding from the mouth, nose or ears.**

WHAT TO DO

- **Get medical help immediately.** Keep the person warm and as comfortable as possible. If the bleeding is severe, try to stop it by applying pressure; see **BLEEDING: CUTS & WOUNDS** in Part One. Avoid any movement which may injure the spinal cord; if necessary, see **TRANSPORTING THE INJURED** in Part One.

RUPTURED BLADDER

SYMPTOMS

Greatly reduced urine output. May occur from a crushing injury, as in an automobile accident.

WHAT TO DO

- **Consult your physician.**
- Treatment may include surgery, use of catheters to provide for urinary drainage.

SPINAL CORD INJURY

SYMPTOMS

Depending on the site and severity of the injury, may include: Temporary or permanent paralysis of lungs, arms, leg muscles above and/or below the knee. Loss of bladder control. Loss of bowel control. Loss of function after a spinal cord injury can be brief if caused by concussion, more lasting if caused by contusion or hemorrhage, permanent if caused by lacerations or a break in the cord.

WHAT TO DO

- **Seek medical aid immediately.** Do not attempt to move or carry the person. As a last resort, see **TRANSPORTING THE INJURED** in Part One.
- Treatment may include such measures as immobilization, traction, surgery.

URINARY DISORDERS

ACUTE KIDNEY FAILURE

SYMPTOMS

Marked reduction in urination. Followed by: Urine smell on the breath. Decreased mental acuity. Other symptoms may include those of uremia; see UREMIA below. Causes are similar to those for uremia.

WHAT TO DO

- **Seek medical aid immediately.**
- Treatment is designed to give the kidneys a chance to recover. May include use of an artificial kidney machine, restrictions in diet and water intake, intravenous administration of nutrients. Consulting a nutritionist can be helpful.

ACUTE KIDNEY INFECTION (Acute pyelonephritis)

SYMPTOMS

Chills. Fever. Flank pain. Nausea. Vomiting. Frequent and urgent urination. An acute bacterial kidney infection, often involving both kidneys. Most common in children (especially girls), pregnant women and diabetics.

WHAT TO DO

- **Consult your physician.**

- Treatment may include antibiotics or other medication, urinary antiseptics.

ACUTE NEPHRITIS (Bright's disease, acute glomerulonephritis)

SYMPTOMS

Fluid retention. Diminished urinary output. Dark urine due to the presence of blood. Rise in blood pressure. Headache. Visual disturbances. An inflammatory disease of the kidneys. Most common in children after age 3, and young adults. Usually follows a streptococcal infection of the throat, sinuses or tonsils, sometimes of the skin or ear in 5 days to 6 weeks.

WHAT TO DO

- **Consult your physician.**
- Treatment may include bed rest, antibiotics and other medication, restriction of protein, salt and water intake.

CHRONIC KIDNEY INFECTION (Chronic pyelonephritis)

SYMPTOMS

May be similar to ACUTE KIDNEY INFECTION with:

Fever. Flank pain. Frequent and urgent urination. Excessive urination during the night. May include indications of uremia; see UREMIA. May follow an acute kidney infection that has not completely responded to treatment.

WHAT TO DO
- Consult your physician.
- Medication may be prescribed. If obstruction is present, surgery may be recommended.

CHRONIC NEPHRITIS (Bright's disease, chronic glomerulonephritis)

SYMPTOMS

Vary. May be discovered in a routine medical checkup through presence of albumin and blood in the urine, with no other symptoms present. In some cases at the other extreme, may begin with: Nausea. Vomiting. Breathing difficulty. Itching. As the disease progresses, symptoms usually include: Puffiness in the face, eyelids and ankles. Abdominal distention. Rise in blood pressure. Breathlessness. A slowly progressive chronic disease, often of unknown cause, sometimes resulting from a mild unnoticed form of acute nephritis.

WHAT TO DO
- Consult your physician.
- Progression is difficult to prevent. Treatment may include blood pressure control with salt restriction and drugs. Also may include measures used in uremia; see **UREMIA.**

CYSTITIS (Bladder infection)

SYMPTOMS

Urgent, painful urination. Excessive need to urinate at night. Often: Scanty output. Sometimes: Blood in the urine. In women, most cases are due to ascending infection from the vagina and often follow intercourse. In men, most cases result from ascending infection from the urethra or prostate, with prostatitis a common cause.

WHAT TO DO
- Consult your physician.
- Antibiotics and other medication may be prescribed. Any underlying cause must be treated.

HYDRONEPHROSIS

SYMPTOMS

Recurring attacks of pain in the kidney area that may

be dull or sharp, in some cases excruciating. May also include: Fever. Blood and pus in the urine. Distention of the kidney with backed-up urine as the result of an obstruction in the urinary tract. The obstruction may result from such causes as narrowing of the tract, tumor, enlargement of the prostate.

WHAT TO DO
- Consult your physician.
- Treatment may include drainage by catheter or other means, antibiotic or other therapy for any infection. Surgery may be recommended.

KIDNEY AND BLADDER STONES

SYMPTOMS

When the stones are lodged in the KIDNEY OR URETER, symptoms may include: Back pain. Excruciating intermittent colicky pain that may start in the flank or kidney area and radiate across the abdomen into the genital area and inner aspects of the thighs. Nausea. Vomiting. Abdominal distention. Chills. Fever. Blood in the urine. Frequent urination. When the stones are lodged in the BLADDER, symptoms may include: Pain above the pubic area. Painful urination. Blood and pus in the urine. Frequent urination. Stone formation is common, hospitalizing about 1 in every 1,000 American adults each year. Possible causes include infection, urinary tract obstruction, gout, excessive functioning of the thyroid or parathyroid glands.

WHAT TO DO
- Consult your physician.
- Treatment may include medication for pain, therapy for infection or other underlying cause. If obstructing stones do not pass on their own, surgery may be recommended.

NEPHROSIS (Nephrotic syndrome)

SYMPTOMS

Appetite loss. Weakness. Malaise. Fluid accumulation, causing puffiness in the ankles, feet, eyes, face or abdomen. A disorder of the kidneys in which kidney tissue malfunctions without inflammation, failing to regulate the water balance properly and allowing great loss of protein in the urine. Occurs in adults but is more common in children.

WHAT TO DO
- Consult your physician.
- Medication may be prescribed.

TUMORS (BENIGN) OF THE KIDNEY AND BLADDER

SYMPTOMS

Blood in the urine. Flank pain. An abdominal mass. (Symptoms resemble those for malignant kidney and bladder tumors; see KIDNEY CANCER and BLADDER CANCER.) Growths may be large or small. Some may have a potential for becoming malignant over a period of time.

WHAT TO DO

- Consult your physician.
- Surgery may be recommended.

UREMIA

SYMPTOMS

In ACUTE UREMIA, symptoms begin with: A sudden drop in urine volume. Followed by: Fatigue. Reduced mental acuity. Muscle cramps. Muscle twitching. Nausea. Vomiting. Yellow-brown skin discoloration. Urine smell on the breath. Itching. Appetite loss. Breathing difficulty. Convulsions. In CHRONIC UREMIA, there is no sudden drop in urine volume, but many of the other symptoms appear gradually. In uremia, the kidneys lose much of their ability to filter out materials from the blood, causing waste substances ordinarily eliminated in the urine to appear in the blood. Acute uremia may result from severe infection, severe burn, injury, surgical shock, transfusion reaction, various kinds of poisoning, drug reaction. Among the possible causes of chronic uremia are chronic nephritis, advanced pyelonephritis, hypertensive kidney disease, diabetes, untreated prostate enlargement, urinary obstructions.

WHAT TO DO

- Consult your physician.
- Treatment may include correction of the cause if possible, medication to relieve symptoms. Dialysis with an artificial kidney machine or other means may be used to give the kidneys a chance to recover or, if necessary, to allow time for kidney transplantation.

VENEREAL DISEASES

CHANCROID

SYMPTOMS

Small painful soft sores on or near the external genitals appear 3 to 5 days after sexual contact, and soon become painful shallow ulcers surrounded by a red border. Lymph nodes of the groin become swollen and tender. An abscess may form. Caused by a sexually transmitted bacillus, Haemophilus ducreyi.

WHAT TO DO

- Consult your physician.
- Treatment with a sulfa drug is usually effective. If not, an antibiotic may be prescribed. All sexual contacts should be examined.

CONGENITAL SYPHILIS

SYMPTOMS

The infant develops blisters on the palms, soles, nose, mouth and diaper area. Generalized lymph node enlargement. Other symptoms may include: A failure to thrive. Pus-laden or bloodstained nasal discharge. Enlarged liver. Enlarged spleen. Meningitis. Convulsions. Mental retardation. Caused by transmission of the infection to the fetus from an infected mother who has not been treated for the disease. Can be prevented by adequate treatment for the mother before the end of the fourth month of pregnancy.

WHAT TO DO

- Consult your physician.
- Antibiotics are prescribed for the infant, mother and any other infected family members. In some cases, the infant may also receive further treatment.

GONORRHEA

SYMPTOMS

In MEN: Painful burning during urination. Pus-laden yellowish-green discharge. In some WOMEN: No early symptoms. In others: Vaginal discharge. Painful and frequent urination. If neglected, gonorrhea may lead to serious complications such as arthritis, urethral stricture, meningitis. In the newborn of an untreated mother, eye infections may occur.

Causative organism is the gonococcus Neisseria gonorrhoeae. Spread by intercourse, sometimes by women who are symptomless carriers.

WHAT TO DO
- **Consult your physician.**
- Antibiotic treatment is effective.
- Sexual partners should be traced and treated.
- Symptomless women who have any suspicion of possible infection should seek medical diagnosis and, if necessary, treatment.

GRANULOMA INGUINALE

SYMPTOMS

Begin with a painless, beefy-red nodule which becomes a rounded, elevated mass. Other such lesions then appear. Common sites in MEN are the penis, scrotum, groin and thighs; in WOMEN, the vulva, vagina and the area between the vagina and anus. Incubation period is from 1 to 12 weeks after sexual contact. Anemia and death may occur in neglected cases. Rare in the U.S.; found mostly in the tropics and subtropics.

WHAT TO DO
- **Consult your physician.**
- Antibiotic treatment is effective.

HERPES GENITALIS

SYMPTOMS

Begin with: Itching. Soreness. Followed by: Appearance of a reddened patch, then blisters which develop into circular, painful ulcers. Ulcers become crusted after a few days, may heal in about 10 days with scarring, then keep recurring. The areas affected include the penis, vagina or cervix, pubic area, thighs, buttocks. Transmitted by a form of the herpes virus responsible for fever blisters on the lips. Develops 4 to 7 days after intercourse.

WHAT TO DO
- **Consult your physician.**
- No cure is presently available, but intense efforts are under way to find effective treatment and a preventive vaccine. Affected areas may be cleaned twice a day with salt water solution. Medication may be prescribed.
- Because of a relationship between herpes genitalis and cervical cancer, affected women may be advised to have periodic checkups.
- Because of the danger to a baby delivered in the presence of active herpes genitalis, special precautions may be needed.

LYMPHOGRANULOMA VENEREUM

SYMPTOMS

From 7 to 28 days after sexual contact: A small blister appears, ulcerates and quickly heals. (It may go unnoticed.) Lymph nodes in the groin enlarge and become tender. Other symptoms may include: Fever. Malaise. Headache. Joint pains. Appetite loss. Vomiting. In women, backache may occur. Caused by one of the Chlamydia group of organisms responsible for trachoma and psittacosis. Occurs mostly in the tropics and subtropics.

WHAT TO DO
- **Consult your physician.**
- Antibiotic treatment is effective.

NONSPECIFIC URETHRITIS

SYMPTOMS

In MEN, 7 to 28 days after intercourse: Mild pain on urination. Usually: Slight discharge containing mucus and pus. Sometimes: More copious discharge. Blood in the urine. Most WOMEN have no symptoms. Some experience: Vaginal discharge. Mild pain on urination. Frequent urination. Pelvic pain. Painful intercourse. May be caused by Chlamydia organisms (also responsible for the eye disease trachoma) and other organisms, not gonococci.

WHAT TO DO
- **Consult your physician.**
- Antibiotic treatment is effective. Sexual partners should be examined and, if infected, treated.

SYPHILIS

SYMPTOMS

About 3 weeks after infection, a painless sore (chancre) appears on or near the head of the penis, or on the labia or inside the vagina. In some cases, the chancre may appear on a lip, breast, finger or in the anal area. If this primary syphilis is untreated, the sore disappears in 10 to 40 days but is followed in 2 to 6 months by: A rash that may cover any part of the body. White sores on the mouth and throat mucous membranes and around the genitalia and rectum. Sometimes: Bone pain. Joint pain. Patchy hair loss. If untreated, this secondary syphilis disappears in 3 to 12 weeks but may return sometime later as tertiary syphilis, which can invade almost any cell in the body and may damage the heart, nervous system, eyes, brain. A contagious disease caused by a spirochete organism, Treponema pallidum. Can be passed from a mother to an unborn child; see **CONGENITAL SYPHILIS.**

- **Consult your physician.**
- Penicillin treatment is usually effective; other antibiotics may be prescribed when needed. The earlier the treatment, the better the chances of preventing irreparable damage.
- Sexual partners should be examined and, if infected, treated.

TRICHOMONIASIS

SYMPTOMS

Typically, in WOMEN: Frothy, greenish-yellow vaginal discharge. Sore vulva. Sore thighs. Painful urination. Painful intercourse. Some women, however, have only a slight discharge; some may be symptom-free carriers for long periods but then develop symptoms at any time. MEN often have no symptoms. Some have a discharge early in the morning; some experience painful, frequent urination. Transmitted sexually. Caused by a protozoan, Trichomonas vaginalis.

WHAT TO DO

- **Consult your physician.**
- Cure can be achieved in almost all cases with prescribed medication.
- Sexual partners should be examined and, if infected, treated.

ALPHABETICAL INDEX OF ILLNESSES AND DISORDERS

EMERGENCY TELEPHONE NUMBERS

RESCUE SQUAD OR EMERGENCY AMBULANCE _____

POISON CONTROL CENTER _____

FAMILY DOCTOR: Name _____ Office _____ Home _____

ALTERNATE DOCTOR: Name _____ Office _____ Home _____

PEDIATRICIAN: Name _____ Office _____ Home _____

DENTIST: Name _____ Office _____ Home _____

SPECIALIST: TYPE _____ Name _____ Office _____

SPECIALIST: TYPE _____ Name _____ Office _____

HOSPITAL EMERGENCY _____ HEALTH DEPARTMENT _____

NEAREST DRUGSTORE _____ Hours _____ Phone _____

ALL-NIGHT DRUGSTORE _____ Phone _____

POLICE _____ FIRE DEPARTMENT _____

AUTOMOBILE TOWING & SERVICE _____ TAXI _____

EMERGENCY SHELTER _____

HUSBAND'S PHONE AT WORK _____ WIFE'S PHONE AT WORK _____

OTHER FAMILY MEMBERS' PHONES AT WORK:

Name _____ Phone _____

Name _____ Phone _____

NEIGHBORS & FRIENDS:

Name _____ Address _____ Phone _____

Name _____ Address _____ Phone _____

Name _____ Address _____ Phone _____

Name _____ Address _____ Phone _____

MISCELLANEOUS NUMBERS:

Name _____ Address _____ Phone _____

Name _____ Address _____ Phone _____

Name _____ Address _____ Phone _____

Name _____ Address _____ Phone _____

MEDICAL INSURANCE: Company _____ Policy No. _____

Contact _____ Phone _____

AUTOMOBILE INSURANCE: Company _____ Policy No. _____

Contact _____ Phone _____

COAL SUPPLIER _____ ELECTRIC COMPANY _____

FIREWOOD SUPPLIER _____ GAS COMPANY _____

OIL COMPANY _____ WATER DEPARTMENT _____

For our free brochure of health care and first-aid products,
send your name and address to:

LIFESAVERS

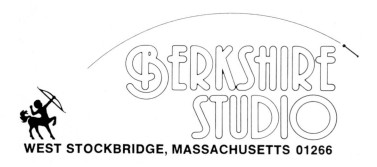

WEST STOCKBRIDGE, MASSACHUSETTS 01266